Healthcare Upside Down

Henry Buchwald

Healthcare Upside Down

A Critical Examination of Policy and Practice

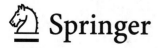 Springer

Henry Buchwald
Department of Surgery
University of Minnesota
Minneapolis, MN, USA

ISBN 978-3-031-07165-2   ISBN 978-3-031-07163-8   (eBook)
https://doi.org/10.1007/978-3-031-07163-8

This Springer imprint is published by the registered company Springer Nature Switzerland AG
The registered company address is: Gewerbestrasse 11, 6330 Cham, Switzerland

DEDICATION: To: All those who require healthcare.
All of us.

Preface

When you see something that is not right, not fair, not just, you have to speak up. You have to say something; you have to do something.
Congressman John Lewis, Address to the United States Congress

The inspiration for this book has been my life as a doctor and as a surgeon who has witnessed and experienced the changes in healthcare and its delivery over the past 60 years. The narrative consists of the history, historical data, and personal experiences about a healthcare system that has moved away from caring, first and foremost, for patients. This expensive system may not be in the best interest either of our nation or of the people it purports to heal.

The topics in this book provide and discuss healthcare statistics and the changing language of medicine. The chapters examine the medical school, the clinic, and the office, the hospital, the practice, the payers, socialized medicine, the underprivileged, public health and pandemics, including COVID-19, and research, as well as the broken doctor/patient relationship. Finally, it offers thoughts on where future healthcare efforts can most fruitfully be expended. These chapters can be read independently, but they are intended to follow in sequence.

I have the greatest respect and admiration for the physicians, nurses, and institutions, which have always been and continue to be the foundations of our healthcare system. I believe, however, that the system has been turned upside down to serve the administrators of the system and away from its basic function of offering the best care for patients. All of us are not getting a fair return for what we are paying. I will provide evidence for this statement by analysis of today's pervading administrative domination of essentially every facet of healthcare.

I hope that this examination will lead us to consider the ways in which we can turn our healthcare system right-side up to serve those who should be the ultimate beneficiaries of such affirmative action—all of us as patients, now and in the future.

Minneapolis, MN, USA   Henry Buchwald

Other Publications by Dr. Buchwald

Also by Henry Buchwald, M.D., Ph.D.
  Metabolic Surgery
  with Richard Varco
  Surgical Management of Obesity
  with George Cowan Jr. and Walter Pories
  Pioneers in Gastroenterology
  with Walford Gillison
  Atlas of Metabolic and Bariatric Surgical Techniques and Procedures
  Let Me Tell You A Story: A Memoir, Volume I
  Let Me Tell You A Story: A Memoir, Volume II
  Let Me Tell You A Story: A Memoir, Volume III
  Surgical Renaissance in the Heartland: A Memoir of the Wangensteen Era

Reviews of This Book

Judith E. "Judy" Heumann

Healthcare Upside Down does an excellent job of explaining the complexity of the US healthcare system that while being the most expensive in the world fails to provide what we should expect as taxpayers. For too long we have been sold a bill of goods that US healthcare is the best in the world while the data clearly indicates quite the contrary. I encourage people in the field of healthcare or just those interested in receiving better healthcare to read this book. Improved healthcare outcomes will strengthen our society for ALL people.

Judy Heumann, author of *Being Heumann: An Unrepentant Memoir of a Disability Rights Activist*, is one of the best-known disability advocates in this nation. She co-founded the World Institute on Disability; she has served as the Special Advisor for International Disability Rights at the US Department of State and has served as the Assistant Secretary of Education for Special Education and Rehabilitation Services. Current healthcare greatly disadvantages the large number of our disabled citizens. Current public amenities and job opportunities for the disabled are largely due to the efforts of Judy Heumann.

Dr. David B Hoyt

This book, *Healthcare Upside Down*, is written from the perspective of someone who lived, taught, and innovated during the golden age of healthcare delivery and patient service. The perspective represented is a true wake-up call about what will happen if we continue as we are without some contemplation of what we expect when we seek care for ourselves or our families and following the values we all hold at the heart. It is written plainly so that anyone in the public will understand the principles and gain insight on how to expand and improve these issues. This is a major work from a highly seasoned professional that may actively help turn things around by calling on public awareness.

Dr. David B. Hoyt was the Executive Director of the American College of Surgeons. Dr. Hoyt was the Chairman of the Department of Surgery and Executive Vice Dean at the University of California, Irvine, before assuming his position at the ACS in 2010. He has championed several major public awareness policies in healthcare, and he represents the voice of organized professional medicine.

Dr. Joseph M. Vigneri

Dr. Buchwald presents a cogent and enlightening exposé of corporate healthcare's emergence as dominant in American medicine today. Even in rural healthcare, the independent practitioner is fading away. Dr. Buchwald offers solutions and challenges. I hope that Dr. Buchwald's book leads to actions to reverse the policies he describes that are detrimental to achieving better healthcare for all Americans.

Dr. Joseph M. Vigneri is retired from private otolaryngology head and neck surgery in rural Casper, Wyoming. His testimony demonstrates that the power of corporate medicine is not only a big city phenomenon, but has extended into the bedrock of American healthcare.

Acknowledgements

I am most grateful to my substantive editor, Emilie Buchwald. She has read every word in this book several times and offered me valuable criticisms, suggestions, and corrections.

I am totally indebted to Danette Oien, who with singular dedication, involving hours of meticulous computer processing, transformed my writing and rewriting into a readable manuscript.

I made liberal use of government agencies and other sources of publicly available published data and statistics.

I wish to thank the many healthcare personnel—doctors in private practice, university professors, nurses, medical students and trainees, as well as the patients, throughout every region of the USA, with whom I talked to substantiate that the contents of this book accurately reflect the current state of healthcare.

Contents

About the Author

Henry Buchwald, MD, PhD, FACS, Hon FRCS (Eng) is Professor of Surgery and Biomedical Engineering and the Owen H. and Sarah Davidson Wangensteen Chair in Experimental Surgery Emeritus at the University of Minnesota. Dr. Buchwald attended Columbia College and the College of Physicians Surgeons of Columbia University. He was the Principal Investigator of the twenty-year Program on the Surgical Control of the Hyperlipidemias, the first randomized clinical trial to demonstrate that cholesterol lowering by his partial ileal bypass operation resulted in reductions in cardiovascular disease and prolonged life expectancy. Buchwald was a pioneer in bariatric surgery and the coauthor and primary advocate of the concept of metabolic surgery. He holds 20 patents for bioengineering devices, including the first implantable infusion pump used in insulin delivery and continuous chemotherapy delivery. Buchwald is the author of over 360 peer-reviewed medical publications and more than 100 book chapters and books. He has served as Co-Editor-in-Chief of the journal *Obesity Surgery* and writes a bimonthly column for *General Surgery News*. The past president of five surgical organizations, Buchwald is the recipient of numerous awards and honors in recognition of his clinical and scholarly accomplishments, including the American College of Surgeons Jacobson Innovation Award (2019) and the Vagelos College of Physicians and Surgeons gold medal for achievement in research (2020). He lives with his wife, Emilie Buchwald, in Minneapolis.

Chapter 1
Statistics

> *It was the best of times, it was the worst of times, it was the age of wisdom, it was the age of foolishness, it was the epoch of belief, it was the epoch of incredulity, it was the season of light, it was the season of darkness, it was the spring of hope, it was the winter of despair.*
>
> *Charles Dickens: A Tale of Two Cities*

A Story

Setting:	**TV Quiz Show**
Story participants:	TV Host, Contestant, United States TV Audience
Host:	Name at least two of the three NFL quarterbacks of all time with the highest career passer ratings up to 2020.
Contestant:	All three have ratings over one hundred. They are Deshaun Watson, Aaron Rogers, and Russell Wilson.
Host:	Correct! You got all three.
Audience:	Response of millions—I knew that! I could have gotten that one!
Host:	When did Dow Jones Industrials first exceed thirty thousand, month and year?
Contestant:	November 2020
Host:	Correct!
Audience:	Response of millions—I knew that! Big day!
Host:	What was Marilyn Monroe's biggest box office hit?
Contestant:	*Some Like It Hot.*
Host:	Correct!
Audience:	Response of millions—I knew that! Too easy!
Host:	United States life expectancy among all nations ranks … I'll accept an approximate answer.

H. Buchwald, *Healthcare Upside Down*, https://doi.org/10.1007/978-3-031-07163-8_1

Contestant:	Not sure. I would say close to the top, within the top ten.
Host:	Wrong! Not even close. It is 40 or lower out of 200, not even in the top quarter of all nations.
Audience:	Response of millions—Wow!

With regard to healthcare in the USA, the quote from Dickens is twice correct. We are in the best of times for knowledge, capability, and potential. We also are in the worst of times with regard to the application of our knowledge and the outcomes achieved, especially when compared to other nations.

The USA has a proud history of medical firsts. We have the largest number of Nobel Laureates in Physiology or Medicine, in technologic advancements, and in the highest quality of healthcare—for certain individuals. At the same time, we are not world leaders, not even close, when we examine the global statistics of life expectancy, mortality rate, potential life lost years, specific diseases mortality, infant mortality, derived amenable mortality to healthcare, healthcare access and quality index, and availability of healthcare.[1] These are the parameters used to measure healthcare and in all of them, given our potential, we are failures, losers in comparison to comparable industrial nations. Yet, we pay much more in dollars per capita and in percentage of our gross national product (GNP) for healthcare than any other nation.

The best way to illustrate these facts that govern our lives is to examine available statistics. In looking at the numbers, it is essential to appreciate their real-life implications. Today's newspaper articles, as well as some scientific articles, will make "statistically valid" claims—by a convention defined as the probability of being factual if something occurs 95 out of 100 times, a criterion fairly useless in the real world. In selecting the statistics for this section, I have used only meaningful real-life data where the numbers represent actual deaths, lives saved, and the quality of life experienced.

Life Expectancy

One often hears the statement that life expectancy at birth in the USA in the past 160 years has almost doubled from 39.4 years in 1860 to 79.1 years in 2020. So, however, has life expectancy from birth in the rest of the world, and the USA is not in the top quarter of all nations. According to the United Nations estimates, Hong Kong, the leading country, in 2020 had an overall life expectancy of 85.29 years (88.17 females, 82.38 males). The top ten countries in life expectancy in 2020 were in order: Hong Kong, Japan, Macao, Switzerland, Singapore, Italy, Spain, Australia, Channel Islands, and Iceland. The USA was ranked below Cuba and Estonia at 46

---

[1] These statistics, and all others in this book, are independent of the COVID-19 statistics, which are discussed in Chap. 10. They are, for the most part, based on pre-COVID 2019–2020 data. Some of the numbers on the tables and figures may be slightly different from current values; however, rankings and implications remain essentially unchanged.

Table 1.1 United Nations Index of life expectancy from birth

Rank	Country	Life expectancy
1	Hong Kong	85.29
16	Canada	82.96
27	Germany	81.88
29	UK	81.77
46	**USA**	**79.11**
64	China	77.47
90	Mexico	75.41
113	Russia	72.99

out of 193 (the US total 79.11 years, females 81.65, males 76.61). The USA ranked 6 years in life expectancy below Hong Kong, about 3 years below our neighbor, Canada, and about 2 years below Great Britain (Table 1.1). The World Health Organization (WHO) ranked the USA at 40th, and the United States Central Intelligence Agency (CIA) Factbook ranked the USA at 46th out of 227 (30th percentile).

Mortality Rate

The mortality rate, or death rate, is defined as the number of deaths in a particular population during a particular period of time, usually calculated as the number of deaths per 1000 or 100,000 people per year. According to the WHO, the country with the highest mortality in 2020 was Bulgaria (15.4), and the country with the lowest mortality rate is Qatar (1.2). There are 227 nations on this list and the USA with a mortality rate of 8.7 is 150th from the bottom (the good end) and 77 from the top (the bad end); in fact, the USA is among the 35% of the nations with the highest annual mortality rate in the world. Annual overall mortality rate has declined over the past 40 years, primarily due to advances in cancer and heart disease therapy, but the USA consistently lags behind comparable industrial nations (Table 1.2).

Potential Life Lost Years

A common statistic of premature mortality is the age-specific potential life lost years (PLLY) per 100,000 population, determined by subtracting the age of death from an arbitrary life expectancy of 70 or 75 years (at the discretion of the reporting agency). This statistic can be applied to specific disease categories for comparisons among nations. According to Health System Tracker, the USA has lower PLLY for all cancers than comparable industrial countries; however, the USA has higher rates for diseases of the circulatory system (including heart disease), the respiratory

Table 1.2 Mortality rate index

Nation	Mortality rate
Singapore	4.4
Israel	5.0
South Korea	5.9
Australia	6.6
Iceland	6.7
Luxembourg	7.1
Canada	7.7
Switzerland	8.0
Norway	8.0
Netherlands	8.7
USA	**8.7**

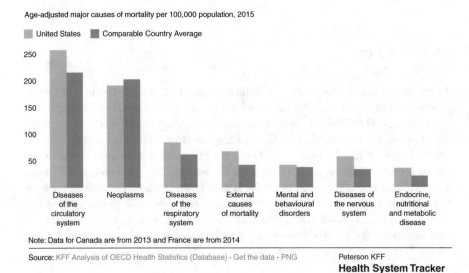

For most of the leading causes of death, mortality rates are higher in the U.S. than in comparable countries

Age-adjusted major causes of mortality per 100,000 population, 2015

■ United States   ■ Comparable Country Average

Note: Data for Canada are from 2013 and France are from 2014

Source: KFF Analysis of OECD Health Statistics (Database) · Get the data · PNG   Peterson KFF
                                                                                        Health System Tracker

Fig. 1.1 Age-adjusted major causes of mortality per 100,000 population, 2015

system, external causes of mortality (including accidents), mental and behavioral disorders, diseases of the nervous system, and endocrine, nutritional, and metabolic diseases, as well as total PLLY (Fig. 1.1).

Infant Mortality

Infant mortality is often quoted as emblematic of national healthcare; indeed, the level of civilization a society has attained. Infant mortality is defined as the death rate under age 1 year of life per 1000 live births. The CIA Factbook ranks 227

Table 1.3 Infant mortality: USA and comparable nations

Nation	Infant mortality *Deaths/1000 live births*
Finland	2.15
Norway	2.34
Sweden	2.45
Australia	3.05
Spain	3.14
Italy	3.14
France	3.19
Germany	3.24
New Zealand	3.50
UK	4.27
Canada	4.44
USA	**5.22**

nations in this category. The three nations with the highest infant mortality are: Afghanistan, Somalia, and the Central African Republic; the poorest score is 106.75 for Afghanistan. The three nations with the lowest infant mortality are Slovenia, Singapore, and Iceland; the best score is 1.53 for Slovenia. The USA ranks 176th from the top (worst) ranked nations and 51 above the best, with a score of 5.22. However, essentially every European country, as well as Australia, New Zealand, and Canada, has a lower infant mortality rate than the USA (Table 1.3).

Amenable Mortality to Healthcare

An interesting statistic has been compiled to rate the standard of healthcare; it is the amenable mortality to healthcare for 100,000 population. This is the mortality that results from medical conditions for which there are recognized healthcare interventions that would be expected to prevent death in most of those afflicted. Differences in mortality for these conditions provide information about how effectively healthcare is being delivered. In 2016, amenable mortality to healthcare in the USA was 112.2 per 100,000, less than achieved by the healthcare systems of Australia, Canada, England, France, Germany, The Netherlands, New Zealand, Norway, Sweden, and Switzerland. The USA is experiencing about 40 more deaths per 100,000 amenable to healthcare than comparable nations (Table 1.4).

Healthcare Access and Quality Index

A comparable index of healthcare is the healthcare access and quality (HAQ) index based on age and risk standardized mortality rates for 32 causes amenable to healthcare. The closer the score to 100, the lower is the mortality rate. The USA and comparable nations have shown improvement in this index since 1990. The gap

Table 1.4 Amenable mortality to healthcare

Country	Amenable mortality
Switzerland	54.5
France	59.5
Norway	59.6
Australia	61.5
Sweden	65.0
Netherlands	67.2
Canada	72.1
New Zealand	81.7
England	84.1
Germany	85.5
USA	**112.2**

Table 1.5 Healthcare access and quality index

Country	HAQ index
Netherlands	96.1
Australia	95.9
Sweden	95.5
Japan	94.1
Austria	93.9
Comparative countries	**93.7**
Germany	92.0
France	91.7
UK	90.5
USA	**88.7**

between the USA and comparable countries has, however, widened. On average, comparable nations saw a 15% increase in the HAQ since 1970 to 93.7, while the US increase was only 10% to 88.7 (Table 1.5).

Healthcare Availability

It is telling to compare the availability of healthcare within the USA in comparison to that of other nations. The number of uninsured Americans dropped from 48.6 in 2010 to 29.3 million in 2017; however, 9.1% of Americans still had no healthcare in 2017. Americans visit doctors less frequently than they do in the Organization for Economic Cooperation and Development (OECD) nations of Austria, Canada, France, Germany, The Netherlands, New Zealand, Norway, Sweden, and Switzerland, with an annual visit to doctors ratio of 4 for the USA compared to 6.8 for the OECD countries (Table 1.6). American practicing physicians are fewer than in the OECD average with a ratio of 2.6/3.8 per 100,000 population.

Table 1.6 Patient visits to doctors

Country	HAQ index
France	5.9
Canada	6.5
Austria	6.6
Netherlands	8.8
Germany	9.8
USA	**4.0**

Table 1.7 Healthcare costs top 15 nations

Rank	Country	Dollars/capita	% GDP
1	USA	10,966	17%
2	Switzerland	7732	12%
3	Germany	6646	11%
4	Sweden	5782	11%
5	France	5376	11%
6	Japan	4825	11%
7	Canada	5418	11%
8	Norway	6647	10%
9	The Netherlands	5765	10%
10	Denmark	5205	10%
11	Austria	5851	10%
12	Belgium	5428	10%
13	UK	4653	10%
14	Australia	5187	9%
15	Iceland	6531	8%

Healthcare Cost

Global statics, therefore, clearly demonstrate that the USA is not the leader, or even among the leaders, in the quality and quantity of healthcare. The USA, however, is indisputably the world leader in the cost of healthcare. Table 1.7 compares the money spent on healthcare per capita and the percent share of the gross domestic product (GDP) for the 15 top nations in 2019.

The per capita (per person) US expenditure of $10,966 is about $3200 more than its nearest cost competitor (Switzerland) of $7732 and 5 to 6 percentage points above the nearest GDP competitors of Switzerland, Germany, Sweden, France, and Canada at 11.0% of their GDP. The USA spends 17% of its GDP. No other country spends over 12% of the GDP on healthcare. The average per capita spending for the 14 nations immediately below the USA is about half of the US expenditure. The average GDP expenditure for these 14 nations is 10.3%, amounting to 58.8% of that of the USA.

Summary

These healthcare comparisons to other nations are offered to present facts to eliminate delusion and complacency, and, most importantly, to illustrate that there are viable goals a nation can strive for. A common healthcare index of value is benefit divided by cost. Healthcare statistics among nations would indicate that the value of US healthcare is far from optimal.

Racial Discrepancy (See Chap. 9: The Underprivileged)

The USA has another problem, namely the marked discrepancy in healthcare outcomes and availability based on race and ethnicity.

Data from the Census Bureau for 2018 shows that the relative life expectancy of Americans differs by race: Asians live 86.3 years, Latinos 81.9 years, Caucasians 78.6 years, Native Americans 77.4 years, and African Americans 75.0 years. The overall age spread differential is 11.3 years, and the difference between Caucasians and African Americans is 3.6 years. The death rate per 1000 is 72.5 for Caucasians in comparison to 85.3 for African Americans. Infant mortality in African Americans is 2.2 times that of Caucasians—10.7/1000 vs. 4.9/1000. Among African Americans, 10.6% in 2018 were uninsured, in comparison to 5.9% of Caucasians. Of African Americans under the age of 65, 12.1% had no health insurance whatsoever. Very similar statistics are available in healthcare for Native Americans.

Conclusions

These numbers are real. The average American will not live as long as the average Italian or Australian, or even as long as the average Lebanese, who live in a country racked by violence. Americans are among the 35% of nations with the highest annual death rate. The average American has, with the exception of cancer, higher rates for heart diseases, respiratory diseases, and most other diseases. The chances for survival to the age of 1 year for an American newborn is below that of every European country, as well as of Australia, New Zealand, and our neighbor, Canada. The average American has poorer healthcare leading to unnecessary deaths when compared to essentially the same "western" societies. The average African American and Native American fare worse than the rest of the nation.

At the same time, the average American pays more for healthcare, and our nation spends more of our gross domestic product for healthcare, than any country in the world.

The following chapters provide and discuss possible reasons for these less than desirable statistics.

Sources

Health System Tracker: https://www.healthsystemtracker.org
KFF Health System Tracker Analysis of OECD Health Statistics (Database) PNG: https://www.healthsystemtracker.org
The Commonwealth Fund: https://www.commonwealthfund.org
US CIA Factbook: https://www.cia.gov/the-world-factbook
WHO: https://apps.who.int/iris/handle/10665/332070

Chapter 2
The Language of Change

Who controls the past controls the future.
Who controls the present controls the past.

George Orwell: 1984

A Story

[After five rings, a robot answers the phone number the caller was given leaving the hospital after surgery.]

Robot:	This is Firm A. If this is an emergency, please hang up and dial 911. Otherwise, listen carefully to the following options: For billing, please press or say 1 [a long list of options follows]. If you're calling for something else, say "something else."
Caller:	Something else.
Robot:	Please stay on the line for the next available operator. Your call may be monitored for quality control and training purposes.

[A considerable pause, with music playing, alternating with an ad for services by Firm A.]

Recorded Voice:	If this is an emergency, please hang up and call 911. Otherwise, please state the purpose of your call for me to direct your call appropriately.
Caller:	It's three days after my surgery with Dr. X. I have a problem. Dr. X asked me to call if I had a problem.
Recorded Voice:	You have a problem after a surgery with us, is that correct?
Caller:	Yes.
Recorded Voice:	I am connecting you with Triage.

© The Author(s), under exclusive license to Springer Nature
Switzerland AG 2022
H. Buchwald, *Healthcare Upside Down*,
https://doi.org/10.1007/978-3-031-07163-8_2

[Considerable pause, with music; human voice answers.]

Triage:	This is Client Triage. Before we proceed, please state your full name, address, date of birth, if you are a current Firm A client, your Firm A client number or social security number, and your insurance information.

[Caller complies with all of the above.]

Triage:	Is your insurance current?
Caller:	Yes.
Triage:	What is the nature of your call?
Caller (sounding desperate):	It's three days after my surgery with Dr. X. I am bleeding. I need to talk with Dr. X. I am also in a lot of pain. Please put me through to Dr. X.
Triage:	It is Firm A policy for me to take your history first. Please describe your main symptoms for me.
Caller (close to crying):	I am bleeding!
Triage (sounding phlegmatic):	From where are you bleeding? When did your bleeding start? How much blood have you lost? Why do you believe your bleeding is related to your surgery?
Caller (now crying):	I am bleeding from my surgical wound. It started today. I don't know how much I bled. Please, please, let me speak to Dr. X. He will understand. He asked me to call if I had any problem.
Triage:	Our staff employee, Provider X, is not on call. I can give you a clinic appointment to see him in three months.
Caller (exasperated):	But I have a problem *now*!
Triage:	I understand. I will refer you to the next available staff provider employee. The provider employee will call you when the provider employee is free; I do not know when that will be. You might wish to go to Urgent Care. If you believe this is an emergency, please hang up and dial 911. Thank you. Goodbye.

This fictional example of a patient attempting to communicate with the doctor is from a column titled, "The Doctor Patient Relationship: Defined by Language," I published in *General Surgery News*, August 6, 2019. The language is an example of "Newspeak" introduced by George Orwell in his novel *1984*.

As a rule, language precedes action; words are the transformative precursors of reality. Dictators know this; reformers and social advocates know this; politicians certainly know this. In medicine and science, every discovery, advancement of knowledge, technology, and therapy is preceded by a hypothesis, by words subject to testing.

The evil world of the novel *1984* is governed by a twisted use of familiar words and phrases to represent the opposite of their original meaning. Changes in healthcare are also dependent on language, and, unfortunately, we have fallen into an era of Newspeak Healthcare that has distorted and is often totally in opposition to the original definitions of healthcare as service to patients.

The Newspeak lexicon of modern healthcare gives common words a new meaning and a new reality. Six such keywords are: *firm*, *triage*, *staff*, *client*, *provider*, and *employee*. Let us examine their common, original meaning, their medical Newspeak derivative, and the provenance of this transition, as well as introducing a new term—administocracy.

Firm (Noun)   A business organization that sells goods or services to make a profit.

In medical Newspeak, "firm" is used to denote a practicing unit of medical care—an office, a partnership, a specialty, a hospital care area, and others. The primary purpose in the use of this term is to indoctrinate doctors and patients into accepting healthcare as a business like any other.

The business of the firm is to be conducted in a business-like manner at a minimal cost to the firm to achieve a maximum profit. Time dedicated to services must be scrutinized and regulated for efficiency and for increasing income. As in all businesses, time is money and is not to be squandered. Time with the sick and needy is divided among healthcare personnel with primary concern for the cost per hour or minute of each practitioner. The most expensive services provided in the shortest period of time (e.g., laboratory tests, X-rays) are the most profitable. Equipment, supplies, and drugs are purchased from the lowest bidder. All ancillary staffing and facilities are administered to ensure that there is no waste of assets. Maximization of profits from this enterprise is, as a rule, not reinvested in providing healthcare nor is it distributed to the actual healthcare workers. Profits go in ever-increasing amounts to the administrators of healthcare.

Use of the term "firm" in healthcare began in the 1990s. While there has been sporadic resistance to this terminology, it has gained in acceptance. This term is key to the language of change in healthcare because its ultimate purpose is to create the acceptance of major change by both the beneficiaries (all of us as patients) and the providers of healthcare. If we accept the idea that healthcare is a business, comparable to any other business (e.g., selling groceries, building homes, producing entertainment), it becomes a commodity. The participants should expect that what was once a personal service is today a transaction.

Triage (Noun)   In medicine, particularly in trauma medicine, this term is used to denote assignment of patients according to the seriousness of injury or the urgency of the problem.

In the evolving Newspeak medical glossary, triage is no longer primarily concerned with the patient's problem, its severity, or the patient him/herself but has become a means to facilitate use of personnel and resources in the most efficient manner in the best interests of the firm. In our dark example, triage is not concerned with the nature of the caller's problem, its seriousness, or who in the firm might be responsible for it. For that matter, triage is not concerned with the caller per se. It is the function of triage to present the problem in such a manner as to minimize the professional time spent on it and to maximize the use of the firm's resources in the most economic manner feasible.

We have all become accustomed to an impersonal business model. For example: You purchase a TV. When it is delivered and installed, it does not work properly. You call the firm from which you made the purchase and ask to speak to the salesperson who sold you the TV. You are referred to triage that tells you that your salesperson will not be available for some time to answer calls, and that someone else will respond to you. However, if you believe your problem is urgent, you are recommended to seek help elsewhere. Eventually, a person will call you, often someone headquartered in another country, who will, after a series of questions, tell you to "reboot" your TV set. Healthcare is moving toward or has arrived at doing business in the same manner, which is managing the health and welfare of people as a commodity.

Staff (Noun) A group of people who work for an organization or a business.

In medical Newspeak, the staff works for the "firm" under the authority of management within a business model of operations. A subdivision of the staff is the service line, a designated group of people within a specialty, for example, cardiovascular or gastrointestinal medicine. Individuals from various disciplines (e.g., medicine, surgery, radiology, etc.) constitute a team or service line.

The egalitarian terms of "staff," "team," "service line" are misleading. In actuality, there is a hierarchy within these units of patient care. In a daily functioning team, decisions are most frequently made by certain of its members, not by the group. This manner of decision-making is particularly accurate for a team containing a surgeon, an invasive radiologist, or an endoscopist, because in the successful running of a "firm," the time of these individuals is best spent if each attends to the special manual activities where the money is made for the unit and for administration. The less-reimbursed medical members of the team, therefore, assume leadership and decision-making.

In certain situations, the reverse is true—all team members are given an equal voice, often to the detriment of the patient and at times antithetical to appropriate medical care. For example, in a hospital "Care Conference" for a critically ill patient that will decide between life-sustaining measures or comfort care only, an ad hoc committee is assembled. Participants typically include the intensivist, the intensive care unit nursing and para nursing staff, a chaplain, and a bioethetician who first saw the patient that morning, as well as the primary care physician or surgeon who has been the patient's principal caregiver. Each person in this group has an equal vote; the primary physician's or surgeon's vote is no more important than that of any of the other committee participants. The outcome of continuing a human life can be decided by a majority vote of these individuals, at times contrary to the opinion of the patient's primary physician(s).

In healthcare, the obfuscation of the terms of staff, team, and service line started before the turn of the twenty-first century. This evolution of words into everyday deeds represents the status quo.

Client (Noun) An individual using the services of a professional person or group.

In the transformation of healthcare vocabulary, "patient" has become "client." This change in terminology originated within the administration of our medical firms as a means to emphasize that medicine is a business. The term "client" entered usage in medical documents, as for example in informed consent, health insurance, and clinic registration forms. At first physicians may have balked at the use of this term, but slowly, over the first two decades of the twenty-first century, the new terminology has become more common, if for no other reason than the necessity to use the word "client" to complete the ever-increasing computer forms in today's system of modern medicine. When healthcare personnel made this transition in vocabulary, patients have come to accept being designated as clients.

The relationship of a medical firm with a client is contractual, thereby eliminating the moral challenge of caring for the tribulations of a fellow human's pathology of body or mind, pain, incapacitation, faith, and hope, substituting instead the concept that the client has contracted the firm for a singular service over a specific period of time for which a fee will be required. When the client accepts these conditions in order to obtain medical care, the client accepts seeing a provider (doctor) not of their choosing but designated at the discretion of the firm at the time determined by the firm.

The client also consents to a team of providers with interchangeable personnel based on the firm's utilization flow chart. The implication of this consent is that there may be a change of the physician seeing a patient, or even of a surgeon during an operation, or of an obstetrician during a delivery. In this contractual relationship of medical care, both the provider (physician) and the client (patient) have abrogated their freedom of choice. Thus, when "client" is substituted for "patient," impersonal service replaces an empathetic relationship and the obligation of one doctor to care for each of his/her patients.

Provider (Noun) A supplier of services.

In healthcare Newspeak, the term "provider" to designate a doctor began to become popular in the 1990s. It was not met with much opposition by physicians, perhaps because they were not aware of the implications of the change, and, that they were in fact providers of healthcare. The term provider, however, comes from the business world, not the world of medicine. The term clearly establishes a contractual relationship to a client. Managing a health problem is the service supplied by the provider to the client.

Further, from the perspective of healthcare administration, the provider designation removes from a physician the aura and prestige of being a highly trained independent professional. Denial of physician independence allows for physician substitution, for physician anonymity, a change that relegates the provider to a cog in the conglomerate of a service line.

Employee (Noun) A person employed to work for wages or salary, especially at a non-executive level.

The transition from doctor to provider in the late twentieth century facilitated the transition from provider to employee in the early twenty-first century. This metamorphosis involved renouncing fiscal responsibility for earning a living and a total transformation of lifestyle for the practicing physician. Yet, the transition was made without much protest. Not only did most physicians accept their new status but many actually welcomed it. Except for some urban institutions and rural practices, nearly all providers/doctors have become institutional employees.

As employees, physicians receive a salary and certain benefits, such as family healthcare, paid vacations, maternal (paternal) leaves, and retirement income from their employer institutions. As physicians, they are free from the time commitment and problems of billing and of managing facilities. As employees, they are entitled to prescribed regular working hours, designated on-call hours, and absence of off-hour emergency calls.

To receive these advantages, today's employee/physicians are willing to adhere to restricted time with each client during an outpatient clinic visit. They agree to having their clients assigned by the firm rather than by client or employee choice, with subsequent care given at the discretion of the firm's scheduling. Surgeons may be told what instruments to use and internists what drugs to prescribe. In fact, the choice of surgical procedures and therapeutic options may be prescribed by the firm. Rules about the use of common appliances (e.g., catheters) are established by protocol. The firm determines how long a client can be hospitalized, whether or not a client should be admitted to the hospital, and, if admitted, to which area and staff. If employees do not practice according to the policies of the firm, they can be severely admonished or fired. In essence, the former doctor, now a provider/employee, has become hired help.

What segment of healthcare was responsible for this transformation both of language and of the reality that followed? It was certainly not the performers of healthcare. Administration changed the language and thus the nature of healthcare.

Administocracy (Noun) The administration of an institution that believes it is in a position of exerting top-down control, based on a chain-of-command structure.

I introduced the term "administocracy" in my 1998 presidential address to the Central Surgical Association following a conversation I had with a university president. He insisted that the role of administration was to lead, manage, and control the faculty, in essence, dictating top-down control, based on a chain-of-command structure. This concept of the role of administration is antithetical to its original mandate, which was to be of service and to assist the faculty. This concept is, however, the one accepted by most of today's healthcare administration. Thus, the term "administocracy" accurately describes the present situation in healthcare.

The administocracy controls appointments, resources, income, and, above all, the employment status of today's provider/employee. By obtaining the authority to hire and to fire, the administration possesses ultimate power. By being responsible for billing and collecting income, the administration controls the money of the firm. After the administration has been generously compensated, monies spent on corporate perks, and on executive search agencies hired to recruit more administrators, those who actually earn income in a medical facility are now the recipients of the trickle-down residue for their labors.

The precedent for the actualization of the administocracy is again a word made into a practice. In 1993, Michael Hammer and James Champy published a book for the business community that coined the word "reengineering." The essence of the book's message is that because knowledge is transient, it is important to reexamine it by starting over with a clean slate, sweeping everything off the table of knowledge, and starting anew. This concept ran a brief course in the business world, which soon recognized it as nonsense and reengineered it away.

In the practice of medicine, renouncing or reengineering the past would ignore the laborious accumulated body of science-derived knowledge. The concept, therefore, gained no adherents among healthcare providers. This was not the case in the realm of healthcare administration. Administocracy embraced reengineering because it allowed abandoning an honorable past of service to medicine for a future of dominating it.

The administocracy has created language to propagate itself. For example, the misuse of the words "leader" and "leadership." In the past, the leaders in healthcare have been the creators and the achievers. The individuals who pioneered a new understanding in a field, who introduced a procedure, a drug, a diagnostic, or a concept, have been the leaders in medicine. Leaders emerged from the ranks of the "toilers in the vineyard" who won the respect of their peers. These leaders said, "follow me," but also paused to help fellow workers. They were prepared, when necessary, to do what is right, even at personal risk. There are numerous examples in the annals of medicine where fellow physicians, true leaders, have come forth in defense of their associates who have been falsely accused of a misdeed, only to suffer adverse consequences themselves. There are also innumerable examples of true medical leaders who spoke out on what was right on moral grounds and their obligation as purveyors of healthcare.

The administocracy today is medicine's ruling class. They view leadership as separate from patient care, research, and public health. They erect a wall between administrators and the actual workers in healthcare. Dialogue is limited to those within their own ranks, while communication with workers is conducted by missives, bulletins, updates, and pronouncements. This transition of authority has been referred to as, "managerial imperialism" (Benjamin Ginsberg; *The Fall of the Faculty*).

Again, language is important. Documents from the administocracy have the aura of orders to the troops emanating from "The Leadership" or from "Senior Leadership." These missives may in fact represent the decisions of a single "Leader."

Several university medical schools have actually instituted "Leadership Academies" with courses for faculty and students. The administocracy selects the candidates for these activities; these courses are often not listed in the curriculum of the medical school. A stated purpose for one such activity is "to create a cohort of early to mid-career MDs from various disciplines to have time to think through complex issues arising in modern health care systems and to form life-long bonds and support for each other as they progress through their careers." In other words—to establish an elitist cadre to govern healthcare and to supervise other physicians. The ultimate purpose of these leadership groups is to maintain and perpetuate the ranks of administocracy as indoctrinated members of a privileged group.

Interestingly, the special training in healthcare this select group receives often does not consist of understanding statistics, complex medical technology, research perspectives, or humane patient management. Instead, the curriculum emphasizes the principles of appearance: how to dress, stand, talk, and write as "leaders." This concept of leadership training is not based on doing but on assuming authority. In contrast, I do not believe that the world's Nobel Laureates and the men and women who built the foundations of healthcare ever spent time learning to assume the mantle of leadership without earning it, to be actors without substance.

Conclusions

Medical Newspeak has normalized thinking about healthcare as a business, a commodity based on cost efficiency. Leadership has been assumed by an administocracy, and physicians have been relegated to revenue-providing assets within a system that processes clients to achieve maximum income for the firm.

Healthcare Newspeak with its distortion of vocabulary has become reality; its functional applications have become, or are becoming, reality. Words matter.

Sources

Buchwald H. CSA presidential address: a clash of cultures – personal autonomy versus corporate bondage. Surgery. 1998;124(4):595–603.
Buchwald H. The doctor patient relationship: defined by language. Gen Surg News. 2019. Column, p 1.
Hammer M, Champy J. Reengineering the corporation. New York: Harper Collins; 1993.
Orwell G. 1984. London: Secker & Warberg; 1949.

Chapter 3
The Medical School

> *Wherever the art of medicine is loved, there is also a love of humanity.*
>
> *Hippocrates, Hippocratic Corpus*
>
> *The concept of a medical school is sacred; its temporary governing body is not.*
>
> *Richard L. Varco, MD, PhD, Professor and Educator*

A Story

A senior professor in a department previously known for its achievements became concerned with the decline of medical teaching, and, having suggestions for remedies, attempted to meet with the dean. The dean's personal assistant told the professor that the dean was too busy to meet with him and asked the professor to put his thoughts into an email. The professor complied and, having done so, asked again for a personal interview with the dean over the next several weeks. In response the dean referred the professor to an associate dean. The professor and the associate dean met several times; the professor made known his concerns. Apart from some minor personal issues, none of the professor's concerns for the department was addressed or remedied. The associate dean, however, arranged for a 15-min audience with the dean.

At the appointed time, the professor and the associate dean were ushered into the dean's office. The dean was waiting for them at the head of his conference table. Though junior to the professor in years and in university service, as well as inferior to the professor in professional accomplishments, the dean kept his hands at his side and made no gesture to offer a handshake or to accept one. He asked the professor to sit. The professor expressed his concerns. The dean listened with essentially no comment for 15 minutes, then rose, and again made no collegial gesture of a handshake, and departed. There was no follow-up from the dean through any means of communication. The professor's concerns remained unaddressed. The associate dean confided that they would not be. The professor had had his 15 minutes with the dean.

© The Author(s), under exclusive license to Springer Nature Switzerland AG 2022
H. Buchwald, *Healthcare Upside Down*,
https://doi.org/10.1007/978-3-031-07163-8_3

This fact-based story illustrates a growing ascendency in our nation's medical schools, the institutions responsible for the origins of our healthcare, of administocracy, of "managerial imperialism," coupled with the decline of the teaching role of the faculty, and, ultimately, a negative impact on the education of our future doctors. A chain-of-command structure and the expectation of rank-based obedience while suitable for the military are antithetical to academia. In contrast, the great universities of the past (and even some of the present) advocated freedom of faculty thought and speech, with administration serving as facilitators for the work of the faculty. This chapter will explore the history of medical schools, their mission, the principles by which they have functioned, and the corruption of these goals presently taking place.

Medical School Origins

Healthcare starts with the doctor. Where does the doctor learn to be a doctor? Who teaches an aspiring physician the trade of medicine, the profession of being a healer?

In the beginning, the secrets of diagnosis and therapy were passed on by practitioners of the art to their students, knowledge often kept within families or special social castes. The oldest recorded school of medicine was established in the ninth century, the Schola Medica Salernitana in Salerno, Italy; it was closed in 1811. Medical schools started to flourish in Europe in the fourteenth to sixteenth centuries, primarily in Italy and in Germany. The first medical school in the USA was inaugurated in 1765 at the College of Philadelphia, as the College of Philadelphia Department of Medicine; in 2011, after several name changes, the school took the name of the University of Pennsylvania's Perelman Medical School.

The mission and curriculum of today's US medical schools are to a great extent based on the book-length Flexner Report compiled and written by Abraham Flexner in 1910, underwritten by the Carnegie Foundation. Flexner personally visited every one of the 155 medical schools then in existence. His critical assessment totally altered medical teaching by increasing medical school admission prerequisites, training physicians in scientifically documented practice, fostering research, giving medical schools control of teaching in designated hospitals, appointing fulltime medical school professors, and strengthening regulations for medical licensure. He admired and was greatly influenced by the Germanic approach to medicine. Flexner was not a doctor; he was a teacher. He was born and lived his life in Kentucky.

The Flexner Report was supplemented in 2010 by a monograph written by David Irby and Molly Cook: *Educating Physicians: A Call for Reforming of Medical School and Residency.* This report emphasized standardization of the learning outcomes and individualization of the learning process, integration of formal knowledge and clinical experience, development of habits of inquiry and innovation, and focus on professional identity formation.

Unfortunately, many aspects of the Flexner Report and the Irby and Cook recommendations, including the principles of freedom of expression of thought and originality, have been subordinated in the twenty-first century to reigning administocracies. Numerous medical schools today represent the aspirations of the administrators for their self-perpetuation as the unquestioned ruling body of the institution.

The Medical School: Mission and Reality

The training of a physician after college consists of 4 years of medical school, followed by residency and fellowship for up to an additional 7 years, licensure, and certification. A modern medical school and its affiliated hospitals have three interlocking missions: to teach the next generation of doctors, to provide the very best of current medical practice, and to engender research and knowledge to enrich the future of healthcare. Let us examine each of these aspects, in particular as they relate to physician training, as to what they should be, what they have become, and what they are trending toward.

Teaching

What makes a teaching school exceptional? Textbooks, libraries, and above all, today's online resources, are available anywhere, but the factor that makes the critical difference between the average and the exceptional is the caliber of the teachers and the time dedicated to teaching. Western society has revered great teachers. In medicine the teachings of the Greek physician Hippocrates have been venerated by subsequent generations. The anatomic lessons of Galen and Vesalius lasted for centuries. Avicenna and Maimonides are often cited as the medieval physician forerunners of medical practice. In more modern times, great teachers of medicine include William Osler, Ignaz Semmelweis, Joseph Lister, Edward Jenner, and Harvey Cushing.

My own great teachers included Owen H. Wangensteen, creator of incorporating the basic sciences and research into the training of surgeons, and life-saving therapy for bowel obstruction; Richard L. Varco, pioneer heart surgeon and originator of metabolic/bariatric surgery for obesity; C. Walton Lillehei, referred to as the Father of Open Heart Surgery, all from the University of Minnesota, as well as Robert F. Loeb of Columbia University, a great mentor of internal medicine.

Though we revere these giants, in their day nearly all faced tremendous opposition, threats, and sometimes punishment. Semmelweis' advocacy for handwashing to avoid transmission of infections was ridiculed, and he was ostracized; Joseph Lister, originator of antiseptic surgery was mocked for propagating the germ theory; Walt Lillehei and Richard Varco were subjected to vitriol and marked opposition to performing their first cases curing congenital heart disease in children. Greatness commonly involves advocating change and challenging the status quo.

There are only a few medical school teachers who will have this kind of global impact, but nearly every medical school teacher has an impact on the medical students placed in his/her charge. The title of "Professor" in academia is, or should be, associated with teaching. Unfortunately, this primary medical school mission of teaching is today often not adequately fulfilled.

Teaching Primary Care

US News and World Report annually ranks medical schools in several categories. In 2021, the ten best schools for teaching primary care are listed as: University of North Carolina, Chapel Hill; University of California, San Francisco; University of Washington, Seattle; Baylor College of Medicine, Houston; University of Michigan, Ann Arbor; University of Virginia, Charlottesville; Oregon Health and Science, Portland; University of California, Davis; University of Colorado, Aurora; and Harvard University, Boston. Geographic distribution: 5 in the West, 3 in the South, 2 in the Central, and 1 in the East.

Though teaching the basic sciences (anatomy, physiology, biochemistry, bacteriology, etc.) may have remained unaffected in the medical school curriculum, teaching the clinical crafts has been radically altered. Time dedicated to bedside teaching has been deemphasized and has become a secondary, minor task for professors. Why? Because the administocracy that rules their incomes, time, and, when not protected by tenure, their jobs, has ruled that the time of clinical professors is better spent in earning dollars to support the pyramid of CEOs and deans with their cadre of associate deans, assistant deans, and their equivalents in healthcare facilities run by a CEO.

Clinical teachers have become employees of the "firm," subject to the time allotments and constraints of the firm's administrative body. In acquiescence to this change in status, medical school professors/teachers have lost their independence and cannot fulfill their sworn Hippocratic oath to provide for the next generation of healers.

I have talked with colleagues in medical schools throughout the country and have been informed that this deterioration of clinical teaching is essentially universal in the USA. There are few fortunate institutions that have not yet succumbed to this trend, while many others are heading in that direction.

The dereliction of clinical teaching in today's medical schools must, of course, have the greatest influence on the medical students—women and men who have worked extremely hard to obtain the college grades and other qualifications to participate in the highly selective process that leads to training for their chosen profession. Students apply to medical schools with great expectations. As a professor, and in the past, the head of internship and residency programs, I have talked with numerous college and medical students about their reasons for choosing a medical school or an institution for post-doctoral residency training. Their choices were based on the national reputation of the medical school or hospital, the learning opportunities offered, and, often on the presence of distinguished physicians and educators as faculty. Never have I heard a future doctor or medical specialist state that their choice was based on the institution's administration. Yet, once they chose an institution, students and trainees enter a world where the dean and the administocracy of the institution determine her/his education for patient care, for research, and, for those who will be in charge of their profession.

As a medical student's education progresses, the emphasis becomes focused on patients—contact with people who are sick, need surgery, have a problem, or are seeking advice. Teaching clinical medicine is the responsibility of the clinical medical faculty. Learning by the students is primarily the result of observation. Too often, today, what the students observe is lack of a mutually receptive, trust-based relationship by their mentors with the patients in their care. They see their teacher's failure to accept personal responsibility, failure to assume ownership for the welfare of individual patients. They experience the interchangeability of physicians based on administrative assignment and designated hours. In essence, in their training, they are introduced to the depersonalization of patient care and the concept that medicine is a business. The outcome of this teaching exposure to "modern" medicine will become manifest in the following chapters dedicated to clinical practice, hospitals, and, above all, the doctor/patient relationship.

Yet, I still hope that clinical teaching in medical schools can instill joy in the process—joy in our profession, joy in learning, joy in helping patients. In their future careers, the joy of practicing medicine may come from time in the operating room, the endoscopy or arteriography suite, the clinic, teaching at bedside, conducting research, writing about discoveries. All are aspects of taking joy in the work. When the work of the aspiring and the mature physician brings joy, the hours dedicated to this work are not a burden. Taking joy in the process sweeps away fatigue and disappointments. In our medical schools, joy in the process cannot be a didactic discipline. It has to be learned by emulation of and from the example set by the teachers and practitioners of medicine, the chosen calling of the medical students and their mentors.

A statement on a person's calling by Martin Luther King, Jr. is appropriate to this discussion:

> If a man is called to be a street sweeper, he should sweep streets even as a Michelangelo painted, or Beethoven composed music or Shakespeare wrote poetry. He should sweep streets so well that all the hosts of heaven and earth will pause to say, here lives a great street sweeper who did his job well.

Yet, within the current medical school climate, there is continuous talk of "burnout," a term becoming more frequent in medical circles. Burnout, defined as job-induced emotional exhaustion, has been a hot topic in analyses of healthcare workers. In 2013, a systematic review of burnout in medical school students was published by Ishak et al. Using various questionnaires as instruments of assessment, the authors calculated that at least 50% of all medical students may be afflicted with the attributes of burnout. How can this be? They are privileged by selection, studying in a privileged atmosphere. They have as yet not taken on responsibility for another person's well-being and sometimes their very life. They are not called upon to make binding decisions as to diagnosis or treatment. In essence, they have not yet actually done anything. How can they have burnout? This is a difficult question to answer. Its basis, however, may reside in the atmosphere and culture of the medical school, and in the teaching being offered. For the healthcare consumer, it seems reasonable to ask how we can raise a healthy crop of physicians to serve the American public if half of the plantings are blighted.

Medical academia should not be a kingdom with a monarch, deputized lords and courtiers, a self-serving administocracy, none directly involved with teaching the ethos of compassion and personalized care for those afflicted with disease or the threat of disease. Ideally, medical schools are the domain of talented scientists, guardians of knowledge, and practitioners working toward a better future. In the sacred institution of our medical schools, leadership should be based on deeds, not rhetoric. The medical school must fulfill its primary function of educating and train-ing of our medical professionals of the future by offering them excellent teaching of humane patient care by clinical practitioners of humane patient care.

Teaching Advanced Care

Various sources provide rankings of the top US Medical Schools, a category largely based on the reputation of their affiliated teaching hospital—the complexity of its patients' problems and the advanced therapies available. On most lists, out of the 155 US institutions offering medical degrees, the following ten university medical schools are the most frequently mentioned: Harvard, Boston; Stanford, Palo Alto; Johns Hopkins, Baltimore; Columbia, New York; University of California, San Francisco; University of California, Los Angeles; Yale, New Haven; Duke, Raleigh; University of Pennsylvania, Philadelphia; and University of Washington, Seattle. The geographic distribution: 4 in the East, 4 in the West, 2 in the South, 0 in the Central. Not quite in the top ten but receiving notable mentions are the University of Michigan, Ann Arbor and the Mayo Clinic, Rochester, two institutions located in the central part of the USA. Thus, the advanced care teaching medical schools and hospitals are fairly evenly distributed throughout the nation.

These facilities have the most modern and expensive diagnostic and therapeutic equipment, e.g., positron emission tomography (PET) scanners, image-guided intensity-modulated radiation therapy (gamma knife), robotic surgery. Their profes-sors understand the utility of computerized "big data," and the use of virtual reality and artificial intelligence to enhance decision-making. These institutions provide medical students the opportunity of access to advanced learning necessary to become the specialists of the future.

The level of their education in the specialty disciplines is, however, once again, the function of the teaching offered by the medical school professors. If the time and emphasis of the faculty dedicated to teaching are limited, subverted to making clinical care income for an overabundant, nonproductive superstructure, the outcomes of higher education in healthcare will suffer. Conversely, if patient care and bedside teaching in the broad sense of that phrase are the prerogatives of a teaching hospital, a higher standard of future healthcare will be assured.

Teaching Research

US News and World Report ranked the ten top medical schools for research for 2021 as follows: Harvard, Boston; Johns Hopkins, Baltimore; University of Pennsylvania, Philadelphia; New York University, New York; Stanford, Palo Alto; Columbia, New York; Mayo Clinic, Rochester; University of California, Los Angeles; University of California, San Francisco; and Washington University, St. Louis. Geographic distribution: 5 in the East, 2 in the Central, 1 in the West, 1 in the South.

Dr. Owen H. Wangensteen, a great surgical educator, believed that every aspiring physician benefits from exposure to research thought and methodology in order to comprehend the ever-changing, evolutionary world of being a doctor. He believed that a vital foundation of the medical school is to offer opportunities for research. Yet today, the principles of research and its methodology are not part of the curriculum of all medical schools. Medical students may be given the opportunity to work in research laboratories, but they can graduate medical school lacking the foundations for properly understanding the rules for judging evidence-based research outcomes. This ability to evaluate as well as to create research requires encouragement by the medical school's professors/teachers who serve as exemplars.

Best of Current Medical Practice

The most current and advanced diagnostics and therapeutics are the hallmark of the top medical schools' teaching hospitals. Their level of patient care provides national leadership in treating the nation's sick. They are the hope, often the last resort, for the advanced cancer patient, the patient with terminal heart failure, the patient with a rare disease, and others. They provide the most experienced patient care of the present, always with an eye towards the future. This essential role in the mission of the medical school, in addition to teaching specialty disciplines to students, must not be compromised by an administocracy concerned with control rather than the ministration of patient care. The choice of new therapies, new tools, must be based on the imagination and originality of the medical school's clinical practitioners, with oversight from a faulty committee, not adjudicated by administration. The business of medicine needs to be secondary to its ethical commitment.

Medical School Research

The objectives of healthcare research are the development of new drugs, new devices, new procedures, above all, new knowledge. The pursuit of insights to prevent as well as to cure diseases and afflictions has received awareness and homage in the modern world. The discoveries of medical research deserve recognition for moving humankind forward on the path of progress. There are government and foundation monies available for providing incentives for researchers, as well as profits for academic institutions. There are also private facilities specializing in research. The pharmaceutical and medical device industries to remain competitive are dependent on research.

The impetus for a vocation in research resides in our medical schools. It is there that many researchers find a home and the financial support and facilities for their careers. In turn, they bring in the research grants that allow the machinery of discovery to function. They and the students they attract add to the prestige of an academic institution, its national and international recognition. Future researchers are taught and trained in medical schools, the third arm in the mission of these institutions.

Costs of Running a Medical School

Over 4 years, student medical school costs in the 2020s were about $150,000 to $250,000. Who pays these costs? Families pay, student loans pay, scholarships pay, student jobs pay, state and federal governments pay, and philanthropies pay. The role of philanthropies is poorly understood and is another area infringed upon by the modern medical school administocracy. One more illustrative story may be appropriate here:

> The Board of Directors of a philanthropic organization with a nearly forty-year relationship with a department of the medical school, and a history of donating millions for research to that department, concluded that their monies were not being used for the resident research purpose granted. The Executive Director of the organization persuaded the organization's Board against taking legal actions. A professor in the department, wishing to preserve this long-time relationship, arranged for an off-site meeting of the Executive Director and the dean's representative. At the meeting, the Executive Director reviewed the current problem and then proceeded, as a member of the greater philanthropic community, to criticize the University on its handling of charitable donations. Suddenly, the associate dean rose and walked out. The only follow-up was a memo from the Office of the Dean stating that the matter was closed and that the Executive Director of the philanthropic organization was never to talk to the medical school administration again or to continue their philanthropic contributions.

Thus, a relationship forged over four decades by generations of people with honorable intentions was abruptly ended. The greater philanthropic community was disturbed; the University lost an ally and considerable revenue; the research mandate of the University was not considered, because a dean took criticism personally.

In a broader perspective, where do the monies that support a medical school come from in the first place? Any family money, old or new, at one time or another, came from services or goods sold to others, as do the monies for student loans, student jobs, and philanthropy. Government contributions come from taxes; taxes come from the earnings of citizens, few of whom have a doctor in the family. Thus, nearly everyone in a nation pays directly or indirectly for the education of its doctors.

Most citizens are concerned about the value of their purchases; are they getting their money's worth? Would the average payer for goods, services, and taxes wish to support the cost of their medical schools? To make this decision, transparency is needed in detailing the money spent for teaching and research, and for administration. This transparency is, for the most part, lacking, and these numbers are difficult to obtain. I would suggest that all of us, the community of payers, are entitled to examine the balance sheets of our medical schools in order to ascertain whether we are getting our money's worth.

Medical School Summary

Throughout this chapter, I have commented negatively on the administocracy that represents an enlarging cadre of our medical schools, in essence, the Dean and the ever-expanding personnel of the Office of the Dean. I have done so because of administration's exerting top-down control rather than facilitation of the medical school mission and faculty. I have done so because of administration's adulteration of the processes of education, of healthcare leadership, and research. I have done so because of administrators who treat faculty and medical school supporters with discourtesy, disrespect, and disdain. The three time-honored functions of a medical school of teaching the next generation of physicians, providing the best of medical practice, and performing research for the future can only exist in an atmosphere of freedom of thought, individual independence for responsible actions, and dreams for contributing to medical progress. For these objectives to succeed, the medical school requires a clinical faculty that leads by example, taking responsibility on a one-to-one basis for the welfare of each patient.

The medical school is the place where most commonly healthcare progress is made. The best of current and the seeds of future patient care most often emanate from the medical schools and their affiliated teaching hospitals. Research and researchers originate in our medical schools. Above all, the medical school is the soul as well as the birthplace of teaching healthcare. Therefore, the medical school must offer outstanding teaching in each discipline, and opportunities for students to practice modern medicine, as well as to understand the basics of clinical research. The success of the medical school in giving each student this grounding will result in creating the benefits and the future of a nation's healthcare.

Conclusion

Another Flexner Report would be useful at this time, an objective analysis of the status quo, as well as recommendations for the future of healthcare, a system that starts in the medical schools of our nation. If medical schools have deviated from their mission, we cannot expect that the practice of medicine and the care of our population will not suffer as well.

Sources

Flexner A. Flexner report: medical education in the United States and Canada. New York: Carnegie Foundation; 1910.

Irby D, Cook M. Educating physicians: a call for reforming of medical school and residency. Monogram: Thriftbooks; 2010.

Ishak WW, et al. Burnout during residency training: a literature review. J Grad Med Educ. 2009;1(2):236–42.

Chapter 4
The Clinic; The Office

In reality most human beings are not, to most human beings, more important than money.

Mokohoma Mokhonoana, South African Author of Aphorisms

A Story

Setting: Two friends talking

A: I need to have surgery.

B: Sorry to hear that. What did your doctor tell you?

A: I don't really have any one person I can call my doctor. I go to a clinic. They refer to themselves as "a firm," and their doctors as "providers."

B: (laughing) I know how that is.

A: I see whichever provider they schedule me with; I still call him doctor. I rarely see the same provider/doctor when I visit. On my last visit, I saw a young one I had never met before. We went over everything, my X-rays and tests, and I was told that surgery was indicated.

B: Did your clinic recommend a surgeon?

A: Not any particular surgeon. They had me make another appointment to talk to a surgeon from the same group. He outlined the surgical procedure, risks, and expectations.

B: Did you like this surgeon?

A: So, so. However, he may not be the one who operates on me. The surgeon I saw made it clear that the firm's surgical group would do the surgery, and when my surgery was scheduled, depending on the group's schedule, I would find out who the operating surgeon would be.

B: I'm sorry.

Chapter 2: The Language of Change introduced the modern lexicon of healthcare, today's transformative terminology governing the relationship of a patient (client) with his/her doctor (provider) in the setting of a clinical office (firm). The

© The Author(s), under exclusive license to Springer Nature
Switzerland AG 2022
H. Buchwald, *Healthcare Upside Down*,
https://doi.org/10.1007/978-3-031-07163-8_4

situation depicted in Chap. 2 is a postoperative emergency for a desperate patient. The daily workings of a clinic or office illustrated in this story is another sad commentary on today's healthcare represented by the current clinic or office medical/surgical practice.

The quote by South African author Mokhonoana is most appropriate here. The clinic or office—the firm—imposes a system of care on the patient—the client—that by billing for several doctors'—providers'—time and services, arranging the time of an operation at the convenience of the firm and not that of the client, the profits for the firm are maximized. These interactions are impersonal transactions. The human client is not as important to the firm as the money the client brings in.

In today's world, outpatient care in clinics and partners' offices has become increasingly impersonal, with decreased physician contact, selection of caregivers made by the organization, key providers of care made interchangeable, and appointments based on a business model, not necessarily on patient need.

I grew up in a city, yet our daily living and contacts were those of a small town. My mother shopped at several privately owned stores: a bakery, a grocery, a fruit store, two different butchers, a poultry and fresh eggs store, a fish store, a delicatessen. Milk was delivered. Each store owner knew my mother, and she consulted them for their recommendations of the day.

We had one dentist and we had one doctor, who was also a family friend. My childhood preceded vaccinations, other than for smallpox. I, therefore, had measles, German measles, mumps, scarlet fever, possibly polio, and frequent strep throats. Our doctor made house calls. He examined me, made a diagnosis, and prescribed homeopathic therapy—cold and hot compresses around my neck, aspirin, bed rest, and certain foods to avoid and others to eat. When he left, my mother had ready for him the expected shot of whiskey to protect him from my germs. For certain diagnoses, he hung a quarantine sign on our apartment door to scare the neighbors. My father, however, still went to work, my mother still went shopping; only I was kept in isolation. It was perhaps not the best of medical care, but it was personal.

Since World War II healthcare has dramatically evolved in diagnosis, treatment, and prevention. Our medical knowledge has climbed astronomically, and technology rivals what was once considered science fiction. New drugs and new operations have become commonplace. Life expectancy has increased and previously mortal diseases became amenable to therapy. At the same time, depersonalization of patient care has gradually increased and continues to increase. Are these trends related; are they mutually dependent? If so, then the end-product of healthcare is manifest today. We conduct some business by electronic communications, hold conversations with robots, and overcome space and time interacting with computerized intelligence. Will the client of the future consult with his/her healthcare firm's computer algorithms for diagnosis and recommendations? If so, the firms would profit; they would decrease their physical space and the number of physicians they employ. If such a virtual future comes to pass, would healthcare regress, be static, or continue to progress?

Depersonalization of healthcare is certainly favored by most administrators of healthcare. What is the perspective of the doctor (provider) toward depersonalization? This is a question I will address in Chaps. 5 and 6. What is the perspective of the patient (client)? The truth is that believing they have no choice, most Americans have accepted the depersonalization of healthcare without protest.

Let us examine the workings of a modern clinic or doctor's office (the firm): The client checks in with a receptionist, the client is given a number, much like in a busy shop or service facility. When the client's number is called, the client is interviewed by a clerk. The most essential part of this interview is establishing insurance coverage, making a co-payment then and there, or paying by check or cash before proceeding further. After another wait, the client is ushered into a room, where the client is given a gown and partially undresses. An assistant weighs the client and takes the client's blood pressure. After another wait, a provider assistant enters, sits at the computer desk, and takes a history; the assistant may or may not do a physical examine. Still another wait before the provider (formerly doctor) enters, at times a different provider than the client has previously seen at this firm. The provider sits at the computer desk, reads the assistant's notes, and questions and possibly examines the client. An expert provider may be called in to consult. Inevitably, a plethora of tests are ordered. A care plan is discussed, the provider departs, and the assistant returns to arrange for prescriptions, follow-up appointments, or scheduling for therapy.

The process is efficient, but is it good medicine? By the lack of continuity of care of a patient (not a client), by a doctor (not an anonymous provider), the actual health problem may not be properly diagnosed, regardless of the multiple test results. The evaluation of the patient's problem may not be appreciated if left to a multiplicity of providers. Prescribed therapy outcomes may lack adequate documentation if dependent on a computer print-out. Above all, no one doctor/physician/provider takes singular responsibility for the healthcare of an individual patient/client.

True doctors think about their patient after they leave the examining room, during the rest of the day, possibly into the evening, and, of course, the next day. Patients like to believe that they can trust their doctor to be thinking about him/her as an unique human who has transferred his/her trust to the caregiver. Group responsibility does not compare to an individual's conscience. Trusting a conglomerate diffuses responsibility and is generally not reassuring to the patient.

In healthcare, the stakes are high. If a client takes a car to a repair firm and the firm does poorly, the car suffers. The client takes the car elsewhere or gets a new car. If a healthcare clinic or office does a poor job, the client, or a member of the client's family, may be harmed, possibly irreparably, and going to another healthcare firm may be too late.

The American public, the ultimate payer for healthcare, has acquiesced to paying for a system forced upon them. Healthcare is as important to life as food and shelter and yet has been made a commodity controlled by the seller, not the buyer.

The average American household spends 4% of its budget on entertainment. Would the average American pay in advance to go to a theater, to a movie, a sporting event, or watch a TV show, if the entertainment venue reserves the right at the time of the event to select the performance, the performers, the sports team, or the athletes? The average American spends 6% directly, and part of the 12% for taxes and 9% for social security, personal insurance, and pensions, on healthcare. The average

American, having paid in advance for his/her healthcare, goes to a healthcare clinic or office and, without a murmur, accepts the venue's choices of providers and provider care. Does this acceptance seem rational?

Paying in advance blindly to purchase quality of life, and possibly the avoidance of death, is a financial blunder. Even more importantly, it is an abrogation of responsibility for the healthcare and well-being of the family. The American way involves freedom of choice. The patient (not client) should have the right to select a person-to-person relationship rather than a mechanized system of healthcare. Can both systems exist simultaneously? If that is feasible, once again the patient should have the personal freedom to make his/her choice.

Conclusions

The outpatient practice of medicine has become depersonalized and is based on the most monetarily profitable allocation of clinic time and personnel.

Chapter 3 concluded that all American citizens are paying for our medical schools and, therefore, should have a voice in the product they are purchasing. Because all Americans are paying for their healthcare clinics and offices, an obvious and compelling conclusion must be that they should have a voice—the loudest voice—in choosing the healthcare product they are purchasing.

Sources

Cayirli T, Veral E. Outpatient scheduling in health care: a review of literature. Prod Operat Manag. 2003;12:519.
Levine DM, et al. Quality and experience of outpatient care in the United States for adults with or without primary care. JAMA Intern Med. 2019;179(3):363–72.
Thimbleby H. Technology and the future of healthcare. J Public Health Res. 2017;2:e28.

Chapter 5
The Hospital

Going to hospital is like going to another planet.

Quenten Blake, English Cartoonist

A Story

I arranged for one of my daughters to have a hip replacement at an internationally renowned clinic by a widely recognized expert orthopedic surgeon. Early in the morning of the surgery, my wife and I accompanied our daughter to the hospital and waited with her in a room in the operating suite. Several nurses prepared my daughter for surgery, placing an IV, etc.; an anesthesiologist came and discussed the upcoming anesthesia events with her; an orderly came for her, placed her on a gurney, and took her to the operating room. The surgeon never came to see us, though my daughter was his first case of the day. After the procedure, my daughter was returned to the room where we were waiting. I asked a nurse if the surgeon would come and talk with us. She said that he had already gone on to his next case. Indeed, the surgeon never came to see my daughter that entire day. Just prior to discharge on the next day, the surgeon spent a few minutes talking with her.

Unfortunately, this story of today's elective hospital surgery is not unique; rather it is ubiquitous. When and why did "provider/client" replace the "doctor/patient" relationship in our hospitals and in our operating suites? The answers to these questions, or at least a reflection on the answers, may be found in an examination of the history of hospitals.

History

Pre-twentieth Century

Ancient Egypt's temples were a refuge for the sick. As early as 1100 BC, Greeks built Asclepieia, temples dedicated to the healer-god Asclepius, where patients were seen and treated by an opioid drug-induced dream, *enkoimesis*, to receive guidance from the deity. In addition, under the same soporific, the Greek physicians performed surgery, e.g., draining of abscesses, removal of traumatic foreign bodies, etc. This tradition continued under the Romans, who also built the first charity hospitals, Valetudinaria, for the care of sick and injured slaves, gladiators, and soldiers.

In the Christian era, the first civilian hospitals were built in the fourth century, starting in Constantinople, capitol of the Eastern Holy Roman Empire. These institutions, called Basilians, included separate buildings for various classes of patients (e.g., lepers), as well as housing for the doctors, nurses, and orderlies of that time. Some of these institutions maintained historical records, funded libraries, and initiated training programs. Certain of these hospitals continue to exist to the present time, e.g., the Hôtel-Dieu (Hostel of God), Paris, founded in 829. In the thirteenth century, the European hospital tradition and construction greatly expanded and gained community standing. During the Renaissance in Milan, portions of the general hospital were designed by the artists Bramante and Michelangelo. Modern western hospitals started to emerge in the eighteenth century, and by the nineteenth century hospital practice was based on scientific concepts, though still influenced by unsubstantiated myths of disease causation, e.g., night air miasma causing cholera.

Institutions created specifically to care for the sick also emerged in the Indian subcontinent in 400 A.D., and probably even earlier in Sri Lanka. Muslim hospitals were constructed in Persian cities and in Cordoba in Islamic southern Spain. These institutions separated therapy departments and divisions by skills and diseases treated. They were also influential in establishing the principle that no one requiring medical care would be turned away because of poverty, race, or religion.

Hospitals in the USA started in 1736 with the New York Bellevue Hospital Center and the New Orleans Charity Hospital, followed by the Pennsylvania Hospital (1751), New York Hospital (1771), Johns Hopkins Bayview Medical Center (1773), and the Boston Dispensary (1796). In the USA there are currently 6090 hospitals, with 919,559 staff beds, including 5141 serving a local community, 1233 for-profit, 962 state and local government, and 208 federal hospitals.

Twentieth Century Transitions

The physical arrangements of in-hospital medical care evolved in the twentieth century into a fairly standard pattern. Entire hospitals, or parts of a hospital, were divided into three sections: ward or charity, semi-private, and private. The large wards consisted of rooms with 12–26 beds, separated by curtains. Financial support for these wards came from the state, the city, religious charities, philanthropy, and to a small extent, patient contributions. The semi-private arrangements consisted of two- to four-bed rooms supported by private patient insurance, employee and union benefits, fraternal organizations, and patient out-of-pocket payments. The private services consisted of single-bed rooms with various degrees of luxury, e.g., a private-patient kitchen with a restaurant-style menu. The clientele included the reasonably well-to-do and the wealthy, celebrities, and mafiosa. During my internship, I participated in the care of foreign potentates, Hollywood stars, and a Broadway composer with a suite containing a grand piano. I was also in the line of fire, but not hit, by a disgruntled patient shooting at a fellow intern.

Responsibility for care was also strictly divided: the wards were usually in or affiliated with a teaching hospital. Care was in the jurisdiction of the house staff, led by the chief resident and senior residents, with attending faculty consultation only on request. This arrangement extended to surgery and the operating rooms where most cases were performed by the house staff without the presence of senior surgeons. The semi-private patients were under the care of a fully certified generalist or specialist doctor of their choice; minor tasks and decisions were shared with the house staff. The same arrangement existed in the operating room; the attending surgeon was in charge and performed the operation, the house staff assisted. In the private pavilions, the attending doctor was responsible for all decisions and care. In the private operating rooms, the surgeon did the entire case, down to the last skin suture; the house staff essentially were there to hold retractors.

It is difficult to say which patient actually received the best care. The ward patient had the full attention of the members of the house staff, who, though lacking in experience, were all eager to learn and to succeed. The semi-private and private patients, on the other hand, had an experienced doctor in-charge; this singular responsibility for patient care could be either the best available or suboptimal.

Until well into the second half of the twentieth century, racial segregation in hospitals was prevalent. In the North, it was the result of "custom;" in the South, it was mandated. I remember in 1956, while touring the Johns Hopkins Hospital in Baltimore, I was struck by the status of their overflowing, segregated wards with patient beds in the hallways. Yet an entire section of a floor was dedicated to toilets. There were separate facilities for doctors, staff, and visitors, each divided into male and female, and, in addition black and white, with the exception of the doctors' toilets because there were no black doctors on staff at that time. I did not see the patient toilets but most certainly they were color coded as well.

When I came to the University of Minnesota Hospital for my residency training, I was astounded by the difference in facilities and responsibility for patient care. There were one-, two-, and a few four-bed patient rooms, all on the same floor and under the care of the same nursing station. The patients occupying these rooms were non-paying, the so-called charity patients, government-subsidized members of Indian nations, patients with healthcare insurance that paid the bill, and wealthy individuals who kept no insurance but paid out-of-pocket. Each patient, regardless of the mode of payment or non-payment, was the responsibility of a patient service. The house staff rotating through that service had no knowledge of who was a paying patient and who was not; they were all treated equally. Each service had one or more attending faculty, who were responsible for all the patients on the service—the patients they had hospitalized for their care, and those they were introduced to on patient rounds. The level of house staff responsibility for each and all of the service patients was delegated by the attendings in charge. This policy extended to the operating room, where a case was never performed without an attending surgeon present. In other words, patient fees did not govern facilities or patient responsibility. Each patient received the best we had to offer, and we, as caregivers, felt privileged to belong to our calling. Regardless of the hours spent in the hospital, we took joy in our work.

Hospitals in the Twenty-First Century

Major changes have been introduced into hospital care over the past 20 years or so. Few came suddenly; most evolved with little resistance by healthcare workers, in particular doctors, as well as healthcare recipients. These changes have altered the profession of medicine and that of doctors, now the providers and employees, who live it (see Chap. 6), and the hospitalized recipients of healthcare, the patients, now the clients. These changes have been initiated and have benefited the ever-enlarging hospital administration, now the administocracy. Above all, these hospital changes have been brought about by replacing the obligation for healing with the business model. With the exception of Veterans Administration Hospitals, hospitals, whether non-profit or for-profit, must be profitable in order to survive and stay in business. By critical analyses, we must ask if the recent changes in hospitals fulfill the healthcare mission, and, if these changes are actually monetarily sound.

Given the business model for the functioning of a twenty-first century hospital, it is important to understand its basis. Third-party charges for services and, therefore, the eagerness or lack of eagerness of a hospital to provide them, are determined by a complex system of healthcare codes. First of these is the Current Procedural Terminology (CPT) system used throughout the USA, originally determined, maintained and modified, and copyrighted by the American Medical Association (AMA). In this system, five-character numbers are assigned to every medical task a medical practitioner provides, in four categories: Category I—procedures, services, devices, and drugs; Category II—performance measures and quality of care; Category III—services and procedures using emergency technology; and Category IV—a subdivision for laboratory testing. Actual reimbursement or payment for services, however, is not uniform but is a function of three factors: (1) The payers can decide the payment offered for each CPT code, e.g., Payer A may pay $100 for a specific code, Payer B $90, and so. The biller can then ask the patient/client for the difference to reach the CPT amount and/or charge a co-payment. (2) The hospital and the payer can make a deal, called bundling, whereby the payer pays a set amount for a particular service (e.g., an obesity operation), regardless of whether the outcome is complication free or not, time in the hospital, and need for readmission. Predictability based on calculations of probability, as in all insurance businesses, is the goal of the bartering parties involved (3). The universal practice of passing on to the customer the expense of paying for the skills of the professional cadres of coding experts hired by both billers and payers.

Of course, Medicare and Medicaid have their own coding system—the Healthcare Common Procedure Coding System (HCPCS), which includes its own Relative Value Unit (RVU) codes, part of the Resource-Based Relative Value Scale (RBRVS), which in turn is based on the CPT codes. These RVUs are a measure of value for physician services formulated on compensation for physician work (52%), practice expenses (44%), and malpractice costs (4%) specific for a particular geographic location. There are several other alphabet soup coding systems, the most important being the International Classification of Disease (ICD) numerology applied by the World Health Organization. All these coding systems are complex, necessitate vast clerical services, and are generally geared to profit the administrators of healthcare, at the expense of the actual income of the healthcare providers, and paid for by the insured public.

Electronic medical record (EMR) systems were introduced into healthcare to provide a better means of managing data and to improve decision-making. With hospitals and third-party payers in-charge, however, EMRs have mostly become billing instruments, and the hospital's information technology (IT) departments are primarily concerned with coding for billing.

Getting In; Getting Out; Getting In Again

Hospitalization is arranged by a physician with privileges at that hospital, or via the emergency room, or some other less frequently means of access. Regardless of the route of admission or the urgency, the first order of business is usually obtaining the patient/client's insurance information or other means of payment. All in all, if the patient/client is solvent, and the hospital has open beds, the hospital is eager to admit patient/clients, comparable to a customer in any other service business. The first day or so of hospitalization is the most profitable for the hospital; the time when laboratory, X-ray, endoscopy, and operating room services are the most utilized, and the greatest number of healthcare personnel are involved. These are the primary money-making days for the hospital.

Subsequent hospital days become less profitable. The need for highly reimbursable services is diminished; insurance revenues have limitations; bundling begins to favor the payer. Thus arises the twenty-first century impetus to discharge the patient/client as soon as possible, and, even better, perform hospital functions in outpatient settings. No longer are post-delivery mothers, or post-operative patients/clients, allowed a day or so of in-hospital recuperation before discharge. After all, their hospital bed once vacated could be occupied by a new customer for those early in-hospital days of maximum profit.

If a patient/client is discharged prematurely, or develops a complication, necessitating readmission, other financial forces come into play. A readmission may be out of the payment zone of the insurer. Thus, emergency department therapy, or admission to a special 24-hour service, may be able to prevent a true hospital admission and its negative monetary income. Another fiscal ploy practiced by administration is admission of a returning patient to a service of the hospital unrelated to the needs of the patient/client, or under the jurisdiction of the attending physicians and the attending's service responsible for the complication. For example, a patient/client with a post-operative wound infection requiring opening of the wound and several days of in-hospital wound care may not be readmitted to the service of the operating surgeon but to a medical service with the specious diagnosis of "fever of unknown origin." Thus, often decisions that should be made on a medical basis with the patient's welfare in mind are made based on financial considerations.

In-Hospital Medical Care

There are still patient/clients in hospital who are cared for by the physicians who admitted them and who may have been their physician for years; there are still patient/clients in hospitals who receive specialized consultative care or surgery by a physician selected by their personal physician; there are still patient/clients in-hospital who have a primary attending physician and a team of house office residents who work with that physician and are there 24 hours a day, every day of their rotation. However, these situations are yielding to interchangeable physicians, physician committees as caregivers, and the employment of hospitalists.

The interchangeability of doctor/provider/employees in the outpatient doctors' office or clinic has been discussed in Chap. 4. The same tag-team care is becoming standard within the hospital setting. Most glaring has been the total loss of patient management authority by the admitting physician, with a replacement physician currently "on-service," someone previously unknown to the patient/client. On some inpatient services, the on-service physicians rotate on a monthly basis; thereby the on-service physician originally assigned to the patient/client can be replaced by an unknown on-service physician when the calendar turns to the first of a new month. In the new world of healthcare, shift work labor has been introduced.

In the past, the hospitalization of a patient was under the management of a senior physician, generalist or specialist, who recruited consultants as needed. Today, care may be relegated to a service line of several physicians. The advantage of this approach is the concurrent availability of various experts. For instance, a colorectal service line specializing in cancer may include a surgeon, an oncologist, an endoscopist, a radiologist, a radiotherapist, a rehabilitation specialist, and possibly others, each playing their part in the care of the patient. The disadvantage of a service line is in the diffusion of responsibility, with no one individual assuming ultimate ownership and the moral obligation to care for the patient.

Hospitalists have changed the performance climate of American hospital care. Many hospitalists are recent medical school graduates, often from abroad, who wish to work fixed hours on a fixed salary. There are two kinds of hospitalists—those who work the evening and night shifts, often in premier hospitals, including academic teaching institutions, and those who run a hospital. The first cadre take care of acute and mundane problems of a service or a designated group of hospitalized patients. Their purpose is to spare the primary attendings from phone calls and patient concerns when they leave the hospital and during the night. The hospitalist is free to call the primary physician for advice. They inform the primary physician of the night's untoward events in the morning. As a rule, this system works well for all concerned, but not always. If the hospitalist commits an error that the primary physician would have been able to avoid, it is, of course, the patient who suffers.

Hospitalists who run a hospital, usually a for-profit facility, rotate on an hourly schedule, do not offer continuous patient care, and accept no individual responsibility for the welfare, life or death, of the individuals in their care. A hospitalist-run hospital fulfills the ultimate business model of healthcare.

Compartmentalization of responsibility to maximize corporate profit has replaced what I believed was part of the obligations of a surgeon, as well as common courtesy. As a surgeon, I have always spoken with my patients before they left for the operating room and made it my practice to visit their relatives or accompanying individuals. I never continued to my next case without first talking with those waiting to hear about the operative procedure I had completed on their loved one. I never left the hospital, regardless of the hour, before visiting each of my postoperative patients.

Restriction of physician judgment can be manifested by the purchase of hospital equipment and establishment of facilities, based on the for-profit, predictability business model. Purchases of instruments, and use of techniques with well-established efficacy, requested by a hospital practitioner can be denied because of cost. In the operating room, and for other interventions, the administration can deny the performance of a proven procedure that the attending physician believes would be best for the patient. In other words, therapy may be decided and in fact mandated by administrators who have not seen, who will never see, and who do not have the requisite training and knowledge to make a life-influencing decision for a patient.

Impersonal patient management is becoming the norm. As a surgeon, I am appalled by the abrogation of responsibility of such a practice.

Hospital Accreditation

The maintenance of high standards for the welfare of patients is a process best served by hospital inspection and accreditation. Interestingly, there is no single national system, comparable to the Food and Drug Administration (FDA), to accomplish this critical task. There are five primary organizations that perform these services, and only one is a federal agency—The Centers for Medicare and Medicaid Services (CMS). The others are: The Joint Commission (TJC), Healthgrades,

Leapfrog Safety, and US News and World Report. The Joint Commission is a national, non-profit that provides certificates of accreditation, rates hospital deficiencies, and counsels hospitals on how to remedy them; it can also remove the sought-after endorsement confirmed by their accreditation.

Accreditation is for the most part an affirmation for achieving and maintaining basic standards. The system, however, by the imposition of specific guidelines can be detrimental. We have discussed the impact of seeking credit for minimal readmissions for complications. On a more minor note, certain accreditation guidelines, such as the number of days to leave in an urinary catheter, regardless of patient need and physician's judgment, are trivial but regularly enforced.

Hospitals: A Business

If the underlying motivation for the current system is good business, why is American healthcare the most expensive in the entire world? If the fundamental driving forces for this paradox are to minimize expenses and maximize profits, where is the money gained going? The users of healthcare pay, directly and indirectly, more than they have in the past, and these costs are increasing, not decreasing. Doctors and other healthcare providers are not profiting; they are making less money, not only by an inflation-rated calculation but in actual dollars. The profits are going to the administocracy of healthcare, the subject of Chap. 7, preceded by Chap. 6 that provides information on what has become of the day-to-day practice of medicine that we, as Americans, are paying for.

Conclusions

In the healthcare upside down hospital institution of today, freedom of choice and loss of authority have been highjacked from both patients and their attending physicians. A calling becomes a job, and a profession becomes labor paid for by the hour for doctors, nurses, aides, orderlies, clerks, and other hospital workers. This depersonalization erodes the joy for the providers of healthcare in the process of caring for patients. This depersonalization erodes trust in the providers and the health outcomes by the recipients of healthcare.

Sources

Carstens HR. The history of hospitals, with a special reference to some of the world's oldest institutions. https://doi.org/10.73266/0003-4819-10-5-670.

Hinchcliff R, et al. Narrative synthesis of health service accreditation literature. BMJ Qual Saf. 2012;21(12):979–91. https://doi.org/10.1136/bmjqs-2012-000852.

The big five healthcare accreditation organizations—a side by side comparison. BHM Healthcare Solutions. www.bhmpc.com

Thomas Craig KJ, et al. U.S. hospital performance methodologies: a scoping review to identify opportunities for crossing the quality chasm. BMC Health Serv Res. 2020;20(1):640. https://doi.org/10.1186/s12913-020-05503-z.

Chapter 6
The Practice

In nothing do doctors more nearly approach the gods than in giving health to others.

Cicero (modified), Rome, 106 BC–43 BC

Success is not the key to happiness. Happiness is the key to success.

If you love what you are doing; you will be successful.

Albert Schweitzer, 1875–1965

A Story

A patient needed a medical certificate of eligibility, a simple summary statement. She requested this courtesy from her primary care physician, a person she had recently seen and who had taken care of her in the past. The doctor readily complied. She sent her a two-line note and a bill for $25.

Charging for a simple doctor's note is an example of the practice of medicine today. It represents a lack of courtesy in the doctor/patient relationship. It may illustrate a lack of independence; the physician is compelled to bill the patient for writing this note by the physician's administration. It may have been prompted by fear of repercussions under current federal laws prohibiting pro bono physician services.

In this chapter, "The Practice," I describe the world of the physician—the doctor, being transposed to that of provider/employee. Cicero's quote, which I have taken the liberty to make gender neutral, provides the ethos for what the practice of medicine should represent. Albert Schweitzer's statement offers a perspective on how to achieve success, applicable to the practice of the physician.

© The Author(s), under exclusive license to Springer Nature
Switzerland AG 2022
H. Buchwald, *Healthcare Upside Down*,
https://doi.org/10.1007/978-3-031-07163-8_6

What Was

Before I describe the present state of medical practice, I will review its past. I take the liberty of illustrating the past by a few stories from my own life.

When I completed my internship, I had a free summer before reporting for my time as a Flight Surgeon, Strategic Air Command, US Air Force. I answered an advertisement to be an independent general practitioner in the Catskill Mountains, where I would be provided with an office, as well as food and lodgings for myself, my wife, and our baby, in a resort hotel, in exchange for taking care of the medical problems of the children in the hotel's children's camp.

I soon found myself extremely busy. My patients included the local population, the summer residents, and the ever-changing clientele of the resort hotel. In addition, the best of the local doctors was recuperating from major surgery and requested me to take his night calls. In my practice, I took care of children and adults, city people whose vacations had been interrupted, local citizens, inhabitants of religious colonies, and true mountain folk who lived in isolation with their pack of dogs.

My most memorable patient was a boy, about the age of 12, part of a family of fruit pickers who seasonally migrated north from the deep south. He had fallen off the back of the family pickup, hit his head, and partially scalped his skull as the family was driving past my hotel office where I had proudly placed my medical sign. The family carried the boy into my office. I ascertained that the acute concussion effects were minimal, and I applied some first aid. I offered to drive the boy to the local hospital. The parents refused, stating they had no money and were not made that welcome in the town. They asked me to do for the boy what I could. I cleansed his wound, gave him antibiotics, an injection of morphine, and sewed the avulsed scalp back into place. I was hesitant to let the boy go to their less-than-optimal quarters and to work in the fields the next day. The family agreed to leave him with me until the next evening. I fed him, made him a bed on my office couch, and, instead of going to my own lodgings, spent the night with him. He seemed to be fine the next morning. He enjoyed the hotel food offerings and was well enough to leave by that evening. His parents came, thanked me, and the boy waved to me as they drove away. I did not ask for a fee. For the next week or so, the pickers moved from peach to apple orchards, and at dusk, the family pickup would roll up to my office door, and a basket of fresh fruit would be left on the doorstep.

I was post-college, 4 years of medical school with supervised patient exposure, and 1 year of actually taking care of patients under supervision in an intense internship, but for the first time that summer, I was alone as a medical practitioner. I made diagnoses. I made decisions. I prescribed and I treated. I tried not to make mistakes and rectified them when I believed I had. I was personally responsible for my actions. I took ownership for the welfare of each person who elected to be my patient. I was now independent. In my understanding of the calling, I was now truly a doctor.

I have always believed that the cardinal attribute, or state of being, of the physician is independence, earned by years of study, hours of work, and personal sacrifice. This independence is costly; it is paid for by assuming responsibility for another's well-being. The ownership bestowed by trust cannot truly be accepted by an entity under the mandate of a third party—the firm, in today's practice of medicine. Servitude is the antithesis of independence.

The sense of the awesome obligation of independence in being a doctor has remained with me throughout my career. After my 5 years of surgical residency, I became solely responsible for the outcomes of my judgment and skills in the operating room, the decision to go to the operating room, and the care of the patient before and after surgery. I was free to ask others for advice, but the ultimate choice of patient management was made by the patient and me. As stated in the previous chapter: I never left the operating room before the essential part of the procedure was completed; I communicated with my patients and their families; I took care of my patients for the full 24 hours in every day. This was my practice as a doctor. This practice can only be achieved when one is free from the edicts of an administrative body. This practice requires independence.

In the past, after residency, and in some cases fellowship training, doctors became independent practitioners or joined partnerships or free-standing practice groups that handled the business aspects of a fee-for-service medical system. The individual doctor selected the type of medicine or specialty they wished to pursue, and the associates they chose to work with. These individuals or groups would then contract with medical services (e.g., X-ray facilities) and hospitals for inpatient care. In turn, the hospital selected those to whom they wanted to grant hospital privileges. Both parties worked together with a common vision of providing healthcare; if their understanding failed to integrate, the parties separated. In all these transactions, the doctor's independence and freedom of choice were preserved, complemented by the patient's freedom of choice of physician.

In the past, doctors performed their own patient histories and physical examinations, made crucial decisions together with their patients, referred or performed the interventions and operative procedures they believed to be the most appropriate for their patients and, in essence, cared for the lives entrusted to them. They did all this without administrative algorithms dictating their decisions. They based their decisions on judgment and experience, with the perspective of treating an individual, not based on mandated metrics of care compiled from majority statistics.

In addition, without extra compensation, doctors performed administrative tasks for the benefit of the institution and hospitals in which they worked and which they called their own. In this task, they were supported and sustained by a cadre of professional administrators, who considered themselves facilitators not commanders.

As for the personal life of the average practicing physician, it is said that they got up early, went to bed late, worked 24 hours per day and on weekends. To a degree this was true. It has been said that they neglected their families and set aside little time for recreation. To a degree, that is also true. Yet, most of us made time for our spouses, children, and other family members, as well as personal time. Most of us juggled obligations without yielding to what is today the common malady of "physician burnout." How did we do this? We took ownership of our decision to become doctors. We pursued a profession, a vocation that gave us the privilege of independence; above all, we took joy in our work. We were fulfilling the admonition of Albert Schweitzer.

One of the tenets of the life of the physician of the past was courtesy: professional, personal, and patient. An episode early in my life illustrates all three of these aspects. I was a medical student in the internal medical service and lived with my wife in a fifth-floor walk-up two blocks from my medical school. It was about 8:00 in the evening when there was a knock on the door. I opened the door and there stood a renowned, senior professor of medicine, professional black bag in hand. He said, "I heard you state today on rounds that your wife was ill; I am here to take care of her." I invited him in and introduced him to my wife. With her permission, he questioned her and listened to her respirations with an old-fashion stethoscope. He diagnosed flu, not pneumonia, and prescribed aspirin and fluids. I thanked him profusely. As he departed, he stated that he was doing his duty as a physician and that I should do the same in my own future.

The precept of professional courtesy for a fellow physician started, as most things medical, with Hippocrates of ancient Greece, and it is inscribed in the Code of Ethics of the American Medical Association. We as physicians are obligated to take care of our fellow physicians and their families without remuneration, a courtesy, a perk, if you wish, within our trade.

Personal courtesy has not been the exclusive domain of the doctor. In that trait of character, he/she is a member of a community. In the world of yesterday, people said hello as they met, stopped to shake hands, discuss the weather and politics. Doctors answered telephone calls and letters from friends, fellow doctors, patients, people they knew, and people they did not know, such as high school students seeking knowledge for an assignment. When doctors walked into an examining room they sat down next to the patient and shook or held the patient's hand; they did not pass by the patient and sit at the computer console. Doctors who admitted patients to hospitals took care of their patients, visited them daily, before and after operative procedures, and made time for serious discussions with the patient's relatives. Medical courtesy was part of common courtesy.

The third aspect of courtesy, financial patient courtesy was integral to the practice of medicine. Providing care for the ill, regardless of their monetary means, began in ancient times and was a basic tenet for physicians until most recently. My granduncle, a veterinarian, a physician for animals, would often waive his fee for treating an ailing cow if the farmer had a bad year, or he would accept a chicken in payment. I did not charge the fruit picker parents of the boy who avulsed his scalp outside my office. In my entire active career, I witnessed my fellow physicians and surgeons treating each patient according to his/her medical needs, not their social position, their insurance coverage, or financial resources. Pro bono service was a moral obligation for our profession.

The code of conduct of essentially every governing medical association emphasizes this principle of patient courtesy. The first 1847 Code of Medical Ethics of the American Medical Association states, "Poverty... should always be recognized as prescribing solid claims for gratuitous services." The fellowship pledge of the American College of Surgeons includes, "I pledge to pursue the practice of surgery with honesty and to place the welfare and the rights of my patient above all else." The Joint Commission Vision Statement reads, "All people always experience the safest, highest quality, best value healthcare across all settings."

What Is

The solo physician or a physician partnership with their own offices and facilities is becoming extinct. With the exception of certain rural and government-contracted physicians, today's healthcare provider works for a large healthcare conglomerate, a hospital, or a business. In essence, most doctors have become employees. The current state of healthcare represents a marked departure from the past, a dramatic change most of the American public is not aware of.

Being a doctor/provider/employee provides the practitioner with a negotiated salary, fixed hours of service in the office, the clinic, the hospital, and possibly the operating room, as well as specified and limited nights and weekends on-call, guaranteed vacation time, maternity and paternity leave, family health benefits, life and malpractice insurance, and a pension. The institution's business unit handles billing, collections, paying office managers, and other personnel, thereby, separating the doctor/employee services from the patient/client's financial status. Employment security is determined by a contract, which generally includes a specified end time, subject to renewal or termination.

On the other side of the ledger, the doctor/provider relinquishes control of the number and the amount of time he/she can see patient/clients, and what services he/she is allowed to offer a patient/client. By altering the doctor–patient relationship to employee-client, the doctor/employee loses individual control of therapy, sharing responsibility with other doctor/employees for the welfare of the patient/client. A hospitalist or other doctor/employee will take management control of the entire group's patient/clients when the originally assigned doctor/employees are not on night or weekend call.

Succinctly stated, by becoming an employee, the doctor gains personal benefits but relinquishes patient control and forfeits his/her independence.

The subject of courtesy is useful in demonstrating the life of the physician deprived of independence.

The time-honored tradition of professional courtesy, treating another physician and his/her family free of charge, is now generally not permitted by the employer institution; indeed, it is against the solicitation laws of the nation. Further, a physician can offer free care to an entire community of impoverished individuals if approved by the administration of his/her institution, but he/she cannot do so selectively by his/her own choosing. If a physician violates this edict against generosity, that doctor can be prosecuted under the federal Anti-Kickback Statute, the Stark Law, the False Claims Act, and Civil Monetary Penalties Laws.

Lawyers working for federal and state governments, health insurance carriers, and hospitals have not only prohibited professional courtesy by physicians but have made it illegal. In contrast, professional courtesy not only flourishes in the legal profession but benevolent and honorable pro bono work is fairly mandatory. The American Bar Association Model Rule 6.1 states, "A lawyer should aspire to render at least fifty (50) hours of pro bono public legal services per year." The New York Bar Association for admission to the bar requires at least 50 pro bono hours annually. This professional dichotomy extends to patient fees as well. As exemplified in Chap. 5, there are price codes for medical services; there are, however, no mandated price controls for lawyers who are free to charge whatever they wish for their hourly fees.

Personal courtesy has not only left the medical world but is absent from the world in general. I have commented on the impersonal nature of communication today in our medical schools (Chap. 3), in medical practices and clinics (Chap. 4), and in our hospitals (Chap. 5). Physician to physician contact has been made more difficult as well, and at times far less pleasant. Telephone numbers are not listed for physicians and, when available, are answered by a machine or not at all. The standard "Hello" today has been replaced by a machine telling you to hang up and dial 911 if this is an emergency. If the robots allow access to a human (in today's vocabulary, a personal assistant), you most likely will be interrogated about the nature of your call and your credentials before being allowed to speak with a colleague.

Finally, and most importantly, in the triad of courtesy, is courtesy to the patient, financial, and otherwise. This aspect involves common politeness, not ignoring the patient for a relationship with a computer, and mandating fees-for-service charges. As has been stated, today's fees are regulated by highly compartmentalized and specific codes. The manipulative skills of the coders and decoders at either end of a payer/payee transaction determine the price paid for a medical service. The physician is left out of this transaction. The physician can neither lower nor raise the charge based on his/her perception of difficulty and time involved. The physician certainly cannot write off a charge; there is no pro bono allowance for the doctor/ employee. On the contrary, as previously stated, pro bono work is legally forbidden. For a relatively poor patient/client with insurance, not even the co-payment can be waived. Indeed, clinics mandate that the co-payment is met before the patient/client can see the doctor/employee. For that matter, all medical services, even most acute emergency room care, must be preceded by the patient/client seeing the gatekeeper and providing evidence of the ability to pay.

With the loss of professional, personal, and patient courtesy, the world becomes a poorer place. Human dignity, nobility, decency, indeed, the very basis of civilization is founded upon and relies on courtesy. The loss of courtesy diminishes us all, and in its gradual, insidious decline, its passing and absence may go unnoticed. In a dictionary of the future, courtesy may be defined as an archaic English term, denoting a quaint principle of the past.

What Will Be

The future rarely plays back the past. However, the future can select principles of the past to incorporate. What will medical practitioners of the future and the society that sponsors and depends on them chose?

Conclusions

In today's healthcare, physician independence has given way to employment and decision management by a hospital or other business entity. This paradigm shift is well exemplified in the loss of professional, patient, and personal courtesy in the practice of medicine.

Sources

Algazy J, Lachs M. Professional courtesy then and now. Arch Intern Med. 1994;154(3):257–61.
Murphy J. 10 qualities that make a good doctor. https://www.mdlinx.com/lfc-2631
Petersdorf RG. Defining the good doctor. JAMA. 1993;269(13):1681–2.

Chapter 7
Payers

Life shouldn't be printed on dollar bills.

Clifford Odets, American Playwriter

America's healthcare system is neither healthy, caring, nor a system.

Walter Cronkite, American Broadcast Anchorman

A Story

(Two women meet in a surgeon's office waiting room.)

A: Do you mind if I ask you if you are here for obesity surgery?

B: No, not at all. I am.

A: Will your insurance pay for it?

B: Well, they made me jump through hoops for a long time. I had to go on certain diet programs for months before I could be considered for surgery. I did all that. Today, I am here to schedule my surgery.

A: I need obesity surgery, I know. I have tried everything else, but my company policy won't pay for it, though I pay part of my premium out of my paycheck. So, after learning more today, I will have to think what I should do next.

B: I am sorry. Good luck.

A: Thank you.

Ultimate Payer

The ultimate payer for American healthcare is us, all of us who pay taxes, have health insurance, and buy pharmaceuticals. As demonstrated in Chap. 1: Statistics—the average US citizen receives second- or third-rate healthcare in comparison to many of the world's nations. In essentially every unfavorable disease statistic, the

H. Buchwald, *Healthcare Upside Down*, https://doi.org/10.1007/978-3-031-07163-8_7

USA ranks higher than every European country, Australia, New Zealand, and Canada, and the USA is among the 35% of nations with the highest annual mortality rate. However, the US healthcare cost per capita is about twice that of most every other nation, with a gross domestic product (GDP) of about 17%, about one-third higher than any other nation on earth.

Are we getting our money's worth?

We pay for healthcare broadly through three intermediaries: taxes, insurance, and directly out-of-pocket. Taxes pay for Medicare, Medicaid, Indian Nation allowances, the National Institutes of Health, and other government-subsidized healthcare agencies. Healthcare insurance paid by employers, fraternal organizations, and other services is paid for by everyone out of payroll deductions, dues, and voluntary purchases. All that is still not enough to cover people's medical needs, so annually most Americans pay out-of-pocket for pharmaceuticals, deductibles, co-payments, and other non-covered healthcare necessities and services.

Insurers

Is there waste in the government/taxes administration? Of course, there is. Is there cheating and profiteering? Of course, there are. But these attributes are relatively minor in comparison to the waste, cheating, and profiteering in the private sector. The public servants of government healthcare in the USA make substantial but not shocking wages. The Secretary of Health and Human Services is paid annually $210,700. The income of the Director of the National Institutes of Health is variable, averaging about $160,000 annually and does not exceed $250,000, about the same as a doctor in general practice in our country.

The payers of private healthcare insurance will reimburse the contracted expenses of the insured for doctors and other healthcare personnel, hospitals, and pharmaceuticals and healthcare devices. The five leading healthcare insurers in the USA are: Blue Cross/Blue Shield (BC/BS) Associates, whose major independent licensee is Anthem; UnitedHealth Group; Aetna; Humana; and Kaiser Permanente. Table 7.1 presents a listing of their subscribers, revenues, stock price, and Fortune 500 rating:

Table 7.1 Five leading healthcare insurers[a]

Company	Subscribers	Revenues	Stock prices	Fortune 500
1. BC/BS associations 　　a. 36 Independent and locally operated 　　　　companies	106 M			
b. Anthem independent BC/BS licensee	40 M	~104 B	~$290	29
2. United Health Group	45 M	~250 B	~$325	7
3. Aetna	35 M	~60 B	~$212	17
4. Humana	20 M	~60 B	~$375	52
5. Kaiser Permanente partial not-for-profit	12 M	~88 B	~$2	42

[a] The numbers in this table are always changing; they are, however, representative of US healthcare insurers

Except for Kaiser Permanente, the stock price for these companies is substantial, and their Fortune 500 rating is essentially in the top 10% of the top 500 companies in the USA.

BC/BS Associates consists of 36 independent, locally operated, companies that offer services in every state to about 106 million subscribers. Some of the affiliates are not-for-profits, others are for-profits. As Chairman of the Board (CEO) of the entire Association, Scott Serota, had an annual listed income of $8.8 M (2017). Of the independent branches, Daniel Loepp, CEO of the Michigan BC/BS, earned $19.2 M in 2018.[1]

The independent Anthem BC/BSX affiliate has about 40 million subscribers, with revenues of $104 billion in 2019. Anthem trades on the stock exchange at about $290 per share; it is listed as 29th under the Fortune 500 companies. The President and CEO of Anthem, Gail Boudreaux, had an annual income of $15.5 million in 2019.

UnitedHealth Group has 45 million subscribers, with revenues of about $250 billion, trades in the stock exchange at $325 per share, and is listed as number seven on Fortune 500. The six companies with higher Fortune 500 rankings are Walmart, Amazon, Exxon Mobile, Apple, CVS Health, and Berkshire Hathaway, all giant monopolies. Walmart and CVS are pharmacy chains and, therefore, also in the healthcare business. The CEO of UnitedHealth Group is Stephen J. Hemsley and his annual income was $18.2 million in 2017.

Aetna, number three in healthcare insurers serves 35 million subscribers, has annual revenues of about $60 billion, sells for about $212 on the stock exchange, and ranks 17th among the Fortune 500 companies. Aetna's CEO is Mark Bretolini and his annual income was $18.8 million in 2018.

Humana serves 20 million subscribers, has revenues of about $60 billion, sells for $375 on the stock exchange, and is ranked 52 by Fortune 500. Humana's CEO, Bruce D. Broussard, earned $17 million in 2019.

Kaiser Permanente serves 12 million subscribers, has revenues of about $88 billion, with a stock price of $2 as a partial not-for-profit firm, and is listed by Fortune 500 as #42. The CEO of Kaiser Permanente Gregory Adams earned $6.8 million in 2019.

The total income of a company's CEOs reflects the success and profits of that company. Salary is usually the smallest amount of the annual total income of a CEO, with the majority of their income coming from bonuses, stock options, and other perks. In the for-profit firms enumerated, the annual CEO incomes range from $15.5 million to $19.2 million, with an average of $17.4 million annually. Of course, the combined annual income of the other officers and board members is several multiples of the CEOs' salaries, quite comparable to incomes in other major non-healthcare industries.

---

[1] The CEO financial data in this chapter are for specific individuals at a specific time; they are listed as illustrative of the monies these positions command. The people in these positions will change. The precise amount of the positions' annual income is not fixed and is contingent on negotiated salary, bonuses, stock options income, and other variables.

Why are these healthcare insurers so profitable? They collect voluntary payments from companies, organizations, and individuals, who must qualify to give their money to these companies, e.g., the clients are screened and often must be free of certain prior conditions or agree to their exemptions from treatment, not be employed in certain occupations, and subject to age limitations or age-determined cost supplements. If allowed into the subscriber pool, premium payments are carefully planned and adjusted by skilled actuaries who are extremely accurate in predicting the probabilities of payouts for disease conditions leaving a substantial overage for expenses, personnel wages, and, of course, profits.

The purchasing of healthcare insurance is usually an easy sell. To acquire the necessary assurance of financial protection from healthcare expenses for the insured and family, the insured feels obligated to join a healthcare insurance plan. In this endeavor, the individual is encouraged not only by the government, but essentially by every well-meaning and responsible friend and advisor.

Insurance premium money goes into a subscriber pool, money goes out to unfortunate individuals in this pool, with margins to maintain the organization. This is the mission of any not-for-profit insurance company. In the case of healthcare, the mission is to provide financial security for the insured to meet healthcare expenditures. Any profit made by a not-for-profit firm, a tax-exempt organization, is usually returned to the subscribers in special bank accounts or in partial payment of insurance premiums.

This is not how the margin of for-profit healthcare insurers work. They create enough profits from the subscriber pool to invest in bonds, stocks, and other financial instruments. If they demonstrate a deep level of profitability, the company goes public with stock offerings, and thereby gains new financial investors in its own stock that then becomes an instrument of growth and further profits. Because disease is not going to go away, healthcare stocks are considered by Wall Street as solid investments.

Healthcare insurance is, therefore, a business; certainly, healthcare insurance is not a philanthropy. This business trades in human misery and anxiety. In these for-profit businesses, the healthcare subscribers do not benefit from a monetary overage; they do not participate in the distribution of profits. On the contrary, if profits are not ample enough for the administrators of the company to maintain and enhance their standing in the business community, additional money can be obtained, once again, from the subscribers, by increasing premiums and decreasing benefits, e.g., raising co-payments, lowering the percentage of covered expenses, and eliminating certain services. The profits of for-profit healthcare companies, in addition to going to administration, are not returned to the paying subscribers but are distributed as dividends to the stockholders, an incentive for the price of the company stock to increase.

Hospital Systems

There are 6090 US hospitals with 919,559 beds, divided into 2946 not-for-profits, 1233 for-profits, 962 state and local governments, 208 federal government, 625 non-federal psychiatric, and 116 others. I have covered hospital ratings for teaching, research, and general efficacy in Chap. 3. None of those mentioned for excellence is among the five top healthcare systems tabulated on the basis of the income of their CEOs (Table 7.2).

The CEO incomes range from $6.6 million to $25.5 million annually with an average of $14.8 million. What is most startling about these numbers is that all five hospital systems are listed as not-for-profit facilities. How can any institution reward their CEOs and also their entire upper echelon of administrators so handsomely, and, at the same time, evade paying any taxes, which is the very basis of being granted not-for-profit status?

If we examine the for-profit hospital networks, the average CEO financial payments are about $six million higher (Table 7.3).

Comparable to the CEOs of the insurance companies, the CEOs of the hospital networks are granted their astronomical annual income because they run a highly profitable business. Whereas a manufacturer of a product, or a service business, must take a loss if the product or service decreases in public demand, the same is not true for hospital associations. They can compensate for potential losses on the books, as well as to bolster their profits, by various transactions reviewed in

Table 7.2 Not-for-profit hospital systems

Hospital system	Location	Number of hospitals and facilities	CEO[a]	CEO annual income
1. Banner Health	Phoenix	186	Peter fine	$25.5 M
2. Memorial Hermann Health	Houston	65	David L. Callender	$18.2 M
3. Ascension Health Alliance	St. Louis	151	Joseph Impicciche	$13.1 M
4. Kaiser Foundation	Oakland	38	Gregory Adams	$6.6 M
5. Northwestern Memorial Healthcare	Chicago	10	Dean Harrison	$10.6 M

[a] The CEOs and their incomes are subject to change; they are, however, representative

Table 7.3 For-profit hospital systems

Hospital system	Location	Number of hospitals and facilities	CEO[a]	Annual income	Stock price	Fortune 500
1. Community Health Systems	Franklin, TN	188	Wayne T. Smith	$6.9 M	~$8.00	251
2. Hospital Corporation of America (HCA)	Nashville, TN	186	Sam Hazen	$26.8 M	~$1.75	67
3. Tenet HealthCare	Dallas, TX	74	Ron Rittenmayer	$24.3 M	~$50	170
4. Lifepoint Health	Brentwood, TN	89	David M. Dill	$25.3 M	~$65	390
5. Prime Healthcare	Ontario, CA	46	Prem Reddy		~$52	853

[a] The CEOs and their income are subject to change; they are, however, representative

Chap. 5, such as bundling care, reducing low-income days in hospital, and only permitting services, facilities, and equipment that are cost-predictable and minimal. If that is not sufficient, in order not to decrease profits, they will lower payment for all the services that they provide, at the expense of the healthcare personnel (e.g., doctors, nurses, etc.), and increase the out-of-pocket payments for their patients.

Pharmaceuticals and Medical Instrument Companies

Healthcare is also dependent on pharmaceutical and medical instrument companies. The top five pharmaceutical companies, based on revenues, are listed in Table 7.4, together with their CEOs and their annual incomes, and company stock prices and Fortune 500 rating. The same information is given in Table 7.5 for medical instrument companies. All these companies are international and for-profit.

Comparable to any other commodity, the sales price for pharmaceuticals and medical instruments is based on the cost of research and development, operating expenses including personnel and facilities, and the profit margin. There are,

Table 7.4 Top pharmaceutical companies 2020

Company	Annual revenues	CEO[a]	CEO annual income	Stock price	Fortune 500 rating
1. Johnson & Johnson	56.1 B	Alex Gorsky	19.5 M	$162	35
2. Pfizer	51.75 B	Albert Bourla	18.0 M	$34	64
3. Roche	49.23 B	Steven Schwan	11.5 M	$42	171
4. Novartis	47.45 B	Vas Narasimhan	14.2 M	$88	225
5. Merck & Co.	46.84 B	Kenneth C. Frazier	22.5 M	$74	69

[a] The CEOs and their income are subject to change; they are, however, representative

Table 7.5 Top medical instrument companies 2020

Company	Annual revenues	CEO[a]	CEO annual income	Stock price	Fortune 500 rating
1. Medtronic	30.6 B	Omar Ishrak	14.8 M	$113	164
2. Johnson & Johnson	26.0 B	Alex Gorsky	19.5 M	$162	35
3. GE Healthcare	21.1 B	John Flannery (Larry Culp)	23.5 M	$12	21
4. Abbott Laboratories	19.9 B	Robert Ford	11.9 M	$123	104
5. Phillips Healthcare	19.0 B	Frans Van Houton	6.3 M	$56	375

[a] The CEOs and their income are subject to change; they are, however, representative

however, two major differences. Pharmaceuticals are protected by patents for 20 years before being threatened by generics, which are often manufactured in pseudo-competition by the same company or by an affiliate. When a non-essential commodity is selling poorly, the manufacturer generally lowers the price to increase sales or abandons the product. The pharmaceutical industry, unwilling to be held responsible for not supplying a healthcare need, will, instead, raise the price of the product to exorbitant levels, causing the buyers, instead of the manufacturer, to abandon the product. For example, liquid Sucralfate, a simple coating agent to soothe the stomach of individuals with reflux disease, has been listed at $210 for a small (14 oz) bottle.

Summary

The Fortune 500 is a list compiled by Fortune Magazine that annually ranks the 500 largest US corporations by total revenues; it is, therefore, a fiscal reflection of the business community. There are over 60 independent healthcare companies on the Fortune 500 listing consisting of non-government healthcare insurance firms, healthcare and hospital networks, and pharmaceutical and medical instrument companies. In total, these companies represent about 13% of the American business community. The revenue threshold in 2020 for being named a Fortune 500 company was a revenue of $5.7 billion. The top ten Fortune 500 companies in 2020 were, in order of rank: Walmart, Amazon, Exxon Mobile, Apple, CVS Health, Berkshire Hathaway, UnitedHealth Group, McKesson, AT&T, AmerisourceBergen. Five out of the top ten (50%) are involved in healthcare.

Walmart, the number one Fortune 500 company for several years running, with annual revenues of about $4 trillion, operates a chain of hypermarkets that include pharmacies and the selling of pharmaceuticals and other healthcare products. CVS Health is predominantly a US pharmacy chain. The UnitedHealth Group has been previously described. McKesson is in the healthcare business primarily as a distributor of pharmaceuticals. AmerisourceBergen Corporation is an American drug wholesale company. Walgreens, CVS, and UnitedHealth together control 54%, over half, of the prescription drug market.

In summary, half of the most profitable US companies derive their revenues from healthcare.

Equilar lists the 100 highest annual paid CEOs at US companies. In 2019, nineteen (19) healthcare CEOs made the list. Number one was Daniel O'Day of Gilead Sciences at $29.1 million, number ten was Samuel Hazen of HCA Healthcare at $17.2 million, and last was Steven Collis of AmerisourceBergen at $11.3 million. Not one of these healthcare CEOs made less than $10.0 million.

In summary, just about one out of five (19%) of the highest income CEOs in the USA are in healthcare. Further, it must always be remembered that the CEOs represent only the pinnacle of the cost of every large administrative pyramid of company officers.

In Chap. 1, we learned that 17% of the gross domestic product (GDP), that is the total value of goods produced and services rendered in the USA in 1 year, go to healthcare, twice as much as any other nation. Multimillions of our nation's GDP, therefore, go to a relatively few healthcare entrepreneurs.

The Business of Healthcare

The data for companies, CEOs (and other administrators), and the GDP clearly prove that healthcare is a business—big business. Is it, however, good business? With regard to company profits, it is excellent business; healthcare is among the most profitable of businesses for certain US companies. But should we not also ask if American healthcare is good for business ethically?

Essentially every American has, is, or will be a patient, need a pharmaceutical, be hospitalized, require a healthcare product or service. The indirect or direct costs for all Americans for the big business of healthcare pay for the CEOs and administrative structure of the healthcare businesses, and is also distributed to the companies' stockholders/investors. There are various alternatives to this business model including these: (1) Make the various healthcare enterprises true not-for-profits, thereby transforming the stakeholders of healthcare, essentially all of us, to the stockholders, allowing us to reduce overhead and lower costs. (2) Reallocate income from administration and stock profits and dividends to pay for increased medical services, lower drug prices, and reduce the GDP for healthcare. These measures become ethical considerations for those who believe healthcare should be universally available and equitable in distribution. In essence, let us ask the question: Should healthcare be treated like any other commodity, for example, the manufacturing of garments or cruise ship excursions, or should healthcare be held to a different ethos?

Finally, it is appropriate to examine the big business of healthcare by the standards of big business. Unequivocally, as demonstrated by the statistics (Chap. 1), US healthcare is turning out an inferior product in comparison to every other first world nation. And US healthcare is doing so at far above the cost of any of its national competitors. From a purely business perspective, can US healthcare survive in its current form? For certain, US healthcare is truly upside down.

Conclusions

The payers of American healthcare by taxes, insurance subscriptions, and out-of-pocket are all of us as citizens. These monies exorbitantly support a cadre of CEOs and other healthcare administrators. Healthcare is traded on the stock market as a commodity and represents a large share of US business ventures.

Sources

Keown A. CEO salaries for the top 20 pharma companies by market cap. Apr 23, 2021. https://www.biospace.com/article/ceo-salaries-for-the-top-pharma-companies-by-market-cap/

Mitchell H. The 7 highest-paid health system CEOs. July 14, 2021. https://www.beckershospital-review.com/rankings-and-ratings/the-7-highest-paid-health-system-ceos.html

Robertson M. Top 15 medtech companies by revenue 2021. Jan 26, 2022. https://www.beckersasc.com/supply-chain/top-15-medtech-companies-by-revenue-2021.html

Walker E. Top 25 health insurance companies in the U.S. Sept 27, 2021. https://www.peoplekeep.com/blog/top-25-health-insurance-companies-in-the-u.s

Chapter 8
Socialized Medicine

Of all the forms of inequality, injustice in healthcare is the most shocking and inhuman.

Martin Luther King, American Civil Rights Leader

One of the traditional methods of imposing statism or socialism on a people has been

by way of medicine.

Ronald Reagan, American President

A Story

A United States film crew was working in Vancouver, Canada, when one of their company developed classical acute appendicitis. His colleagues drove him to the nearest hospital where they were turned away and told that the facility had maximized its quota for appendectomies. The emergency room directed them to another hospital. There they received the same welcome. The film crew next rushed their member across the border to a small United States country hospital where the patient was admitted, operated, and cared for.

Definitions

Single Payer

Single payer healthcare has a dual meaning. The term is used to represent a national universal healthcare system where healthcare costs are covered by a single public payer that may either: (1) contract for services from private organizations or (2) may own and employ the healthcare resources and personnel. An example of the former is Canada, of the latter Great Britain.

© The Author(s), under exclusive license to Springer Nature
Switzerland AG 2022
H. Buchwald, *Healthcare Upside Down*,
https://doi.org/10.1007/978-3-031-07163-8_8

The first alternative eliminates the independent big business insurers and can, by setting pricing, partly control the big business practices of clinic and hospital networks and pharmaceuticals and healthcare equipment companies. The second alternative places total control of healthcare in the hands of the government.

In truth, the definition per se of "single payer" is misleading; the term "public payer" actually means government, and government financing is from taxes. The source of taxes is the citizens of a country. Therefore, "single payer" in actuality equals multiple payers—all of us who pay taxes.

Socialized Medicine

Socialized medicine is a term for universal healthcare that is widely misused. In the USA, the term has taken on a pejorative connotation in discussing any aspect of government-controlled healthcare. When first introduced in the USA in the early twentieth century, socialized medicine was a term of praise for social health consciousness and diversity. A form of national health insurance was advocated by Presidents Theodore Roosevelt, Franklin D. Roosevelt, and Harry S. Truman. Currently in the USA, the rubric of government-controlled socialized medicine can justifiably be applied to healthcare under the Veteran's Administration, all branches of the Armed Forces, the Indian Healthcare network, Medicare for the elderly, Medicaid for the poor, and the recipients of insurance under the Affordable Care Act.

US Healthcare System

Some would say that we have a capitalist healthcare system, a free-for-all, with minimal restraints and controls, governed by the varying fortunes of the marketplace. But by the very definition of the means for success in the capitalist world of big business, US healthcare is a failure. Our system profits only a few, provides an inferior product (Chap. 1), and does so at a cost far higher than that of its competitors (Chaps. 1 and 7).

Many Americans rely on *Consumer Reports* magazine in making their choices. This journal offers extremely detailed analyses tables encompassing nearly every feature of a product, e.g., the acceleration, braking, safety, tires, etc. of automobiles, as well as the market price and a cost/value rating. If the US buyer had the same choice in healthcare as in selecting a car, the buyer would not purchase our current mess of a system.

Are we a socialized medicine nation? We do not believe we are, though 60–65% of our population has one form or another of government-financed healthcare. This circumstance has come about because the big business model of healthcare has failed so many of our citizens, and the Gross Domestic Product dedicated to healthcare is out of control. Some would advocate markedly reducing the percentage of government-financed healthcare to well below 50%; others want to increase it to 100%.

To put it bluntly, the US healthcare system today is an amalgamated shambles.

Principals and Practices of Socialized Medicine: The Good and the Bad

Universal Healthcare

The USA is the only wealthy, industrialized country that does not provide universal healthcare. In other words, all those other nations believe healthcare is an unalienable right, one that cannot be restrained or repealed by human laws, and that in order to secure these rights governments are created. In the preamble to the United States Declaration of Independence, three unalienable rights are specified: life, liberty, and the pursuit of happiness. It is reasonable to conclude that universal healthcare embodies them all.

Equity of Care

Equity of care prescribes that all who are sick should receive the best available medical attention, regardless of their financial status. During my training and active years as a surgeon, this principle was practiced by nearly all frontline caregivers. In some hospitals you could buy accommodations, certain clinic facilities were grander than others, but the patient care was equitable, and, unlike today, select pharmaceuticals were not unreasonably priced out of the means of some of the needy.

The same was true in the socialized medicine countries I have visited in Europe. There was, however, anything but equity of resources and care in the communist version of socialized medicine practiced in the Soviet Union. In 1988, I was selected by the USA to lead a group of 40 surgeons on a goodwill tour of Soviet medical centers as part of *Glosnost* before the dissolution of the Soviet Union. There were general and specialty hospitals in the Soviet Union for the citizenry, but also more sophisticated facilities for members of the Communist Party, and exclusive establishments for the Politbureau. The system boasted of equality, but some were more equal than others.

Exclusions from Care

Socialized medicine stresses no exclusions for care for prior disease conditions. This principle is integral to the US socialized care institutions, listed above. Conversely, US for-profit and not-for-profit medical insurers practice age discrimination, as well as prior conditions discrimination. A heart attack in the past, presence of diabetes, etc. could be the basis of insurance denied or exclusion of any medical problems related to the past, or, at best, the requirement of an extra premium payment. National laws today prohibit exclusion clauses on government-supported health insurance policies; in the private sector, the situation is more nebulous, with exclusions for a set period of time for certain afflictions being permissible.

Access to Care

Any form of socialized medicine or single payer healthcare controls access to care with all of its implications. The administration determines what medical care is offered, what surgical procedures are sanctioned, what drugs can be used. Without the approval of a central bureaucracy, there is no access to care.

A comedic story can be illustrative. The socialized medicine service of Belgium approved obesity surgery as a readily available option, but did not approve the performance of a particular operation—the biliopancreatic diversion/duodenal switch. The excellent obesity surgeons in Belgium, skilled in the performance of the difficult biliopancreatic diversion/duodenal switch, were free to perform the operation; however, the citizens of Belgium would not be eligible to have the procedure paid for. The socialized medicine system of Great Britain, on the other hand, was slow in starting obesity surgery. As a consequence, English citizens with money crossed the English Channel to have a biliopancreatic diversion/duodenal switch in Belgium.

A more compelling example of restriction of access to care by a socialized medicine network is the often cited waiting time for a particular therapy. It is not uncommon for cardiac patients waiting for assignment for required surgery to deteriorate and have their life expectancy diminished. In essence, under socialized medicine, a national government can restrict essential healthcare or deny it for budgetary reasons. This tendency of socialized medicine to restrict access to care is practiced even in countries with a small population such as New Zealand.

Quotas

Another cardinal aspect of socialized medicine is the setting of quotas for particular services, especially operations. There are also decreed budget caps for certain healthcare services; when the annual cap is reached, these services are suspended until the next fiscal year. Once a facility's numeric or financial quota is met, there is no further national reimbursement for that service. If the clinic or hospital facility then elects to perform that service, it is at their own expense, in essence, a financial debit for the institution.

I live in Minnesota where we have excellent healthcare facilities. We have seen, especially in years past, a stream of patients, who can afford it, from our neighbor, Canada, coming across the border for surgery and other therapy because of quotas, as well as denied access to care and exclusions from healthcare.

Patient Freedom of Choice

Under Canadian healthcare, which is considered exemplary of the socialized medicine model, any Canadian can choose to receive care from any physician or hospital, usually within their province, as long as that doctor or facility is accepting new patients. There is no limit to the number of different physicians a Canadian can see. If the individual is not satisfied with the care received, he/she may choose to change to another physician or hospital.

In the US system, on the contrary, for most patients, freedom of healthcare choice is far more limited. The individual patient is limited in his/her choice by the insurance/hospital network they, or their employer, has chosen. Within that network, they often cannot choose an individual physician (Chaps. 4, 5, and 6). Further, they may have no control of a change in physicians or services available.

Certainly, with respect to choice of physicians the Canadian socialized medicine system beats ours.

Physician Freedom of Choice

Under socialized medicine, physicians' freedom of choice is often quite limited. The physician can be mandated to offer, or not to offer, certain services for a specific disease, including medical, surgical, rehabilitation, and other functions of healthcare. The same restraints are being placed on US physicians, who now, for the most part, are employees and not autonomous practitioners (Chap. 6). It is difficult to conjecture whether socialized or the current US systems offer greater liberty, or restrictions, on the practice of medicine.

Preventative Healthcare

Socialized medicine has learned to look into the future and to recognize that preventative healthcare makes for a healthier population, and, most importantly, is less expensive, long-range healthcare. This concept has had great difficulty entering the US psyche. US doctors have traditionally been trained to treat disease not prevent it. Hours upon hours are spent in medical school and postgraduate training on heart

attacks, heart failure, dysrhythmias, strokes, aneurysms, aortic dissections, periph-
eral vascular disease, and other manifestations of atherosclerosis; yet, little time is
spent on preventing atherosclerosis by maintaining low cholesterol concentrations
and a normal blood pressure, preventing diabetes, and avoiding smoking. Only
recently, have proper nutrition and avoidance and treatment of obesity been made
part of the medical curriculum.

Use of Medical Care

It is probably accurate that under socialized medicine people go to their healthcare
facilities unnecessarily with minor problems in the belief that because their taxes
have paid for healthcare services, they should utilize them. I know that healthy individuals in Europe elect to spend several weeks in a government recuperation facility
with free food in the mountains because they feel entitled to do so. There is an
apocryphal story in this regard: Several retired acquaintances agreed to meet peri-
odically in their doctor's office primarily to socialize and review some minor issue
with the physician. One day the doctor enters the waiting room and finds one member of the group absent and inquires about the person. The doctor is told that the
absentee felt too ill to come.

In the USA, the problem of excess, unnecessary use of healthcare ostensibly was
meant to be dealt with by the co-payment system, making the patient pay a certain
amount out-of-pocket to get to see the doctor. It is far more likely that the co-
payment system was instituted to increase the profit margin and CEOs' incomes in
the US big business model.

Quality of Care

Today, in the industrialized world, in the nations with a socialized medicine system,
the quality of care, by overwhelming statistical analysis, is the best available (Chap.
1). In essentially every category of factual assessment, healthcare under socialized
medicine in these countries is superior to that available in the USA. Patriotic rhetoric aside, facts are facts.

Conclusions

There are good features to socialized medicine.
There are bad features to socialized medicine.
Certain areas of the US healthcare network are currently represented by a single
payer, socialized medicine system.

Today, healthcare under socialized medicine in industrialized countries is, as a rule, statistically better than healthcare in the USA.

The challenge for all of us is to fix, alter, improve, create a plan for a new, unique, and humane US healthcare suitable for a democracy that values independence and acknowledges citizen responsibility.

Sources

Bizzle M, et al. The specter of socialized medicine. What is it and is it invading our country? May 14, 2008. https://www.americanprogress.org/article/the-specter-of-socialized-medicine/

Cruz T. Fact sheet: socialized medicine is a failure everywhere it's been tried. Feb 7, 2017. https://www.cruz.senate.gov/newsroom/press-releases/fact-sheet-socialized-medicine-is-a-failure-everywhere-it-and-039s-been-tried

Kersler-Starkey K, Bunch LN. health insurance coverage in the United States 2020. Sep 14, 2021. https://www.census.gov/library/publications/2021/demo/p60-274.html

Torrey T. Differences between universal healthcare and socialized medicine. Feb 27, 2020. https://www.verywellhealth.com/is-universal-healthcare-the-same-as-socialized-medicine-3969754

Chapter 9
The Underprivileged

Things you take for granted someone else is praying for.

Marlan Rico Lee, Musician

A True Story

In April 1977, Judy Heumann and about 150 others staged the longest takeover of a government building in United States history: A peaceful sit-in demonstration of 28 days in the United States Department of Health, Education, and Welfare building in San Francisco in a protest to define and secure universal rights for the disabled. This action pressured the Carter administration to implement mandates that ultimately led to the creation of the *Americans With Disabilities Act* of July 26, 1990, signed into law by President George H.W. Bush.

From prehistoric times forward there have been underprivileged individuals, those deprived of certain necessities and conveniences available to the majority of the members of their society. This chapter considers the healthcare of the under-privileged segments of our US population. There are those who choose not to avail themselves of modern healthcare. As long as that decision does not infringe on the health of others in the community, this decision is their privilege. The truly under-privileged do not enjoy the fruits of healthcare they desire, indeed, are entitled to. The root cause for their lack of healthcare is lack of funds. Poverty is the common underlying cause of healthcare deprivation that springs from race, gender, caste, religion, and having a disability.

© The Author(s), under exclusive license to Springer Nature
Switzerland AG 2022
H. Buchwald, *Healthcare Upside Down*,
https://doi.org/10.1007/978-3-031-07163-8_9

Historical Notes

Ancient Egypt

In addition to prayer, Egyptian healthcare consisted of drug remedies and surgical procedures, with surgery based on a fairly sophisticated knowledge of anatomy. The Egyptians treated gastrointestinal, gynecological, and urinary tract problems, as well as practicing dentistry. They diagnosed diabetes and cancer. Their surgical instruments were the forerunners of today's operating room equipment. They performed circumcisions, sutured wounds, cauterized bleeding vessels, drained abscesses, and splinted broken bones. They produced an extensive papyri medical literature. They had temples dedicated to healing and a hierarchy of physicians. Egyptian royalty received the best of Egyptian healthcare, as did Egyptians with wealth, but many common citizens were not excluded. For example, the major edifices of ancient Egypt, the pyramids and temples, and in particular the tombs in the Valley of the Kings and the Valley of the Queens were not constructed by slaves but by skilled workmen who received medical care under a state-subsidized public health system.

Ancient China

Ancient Chinese medicine included acupuncture, tai chi, and a huge assortment of herbal products and concocted medicines. Most interestingly, these Chinese doctors were more concerned with preventing disease than treating it; in essence they practiced a form of public health medicine. Doctors received a retainer to keep a patient well that was suspended if the patient became ill and restarted if the patient was cured of his/her illness. In this system, those too poor to pay were healthcare underprivileged. (Today, with the institution of "concierge" medicine (see Chap. 13), a similar class of the healthcare underprivileged has been created in our country.)

Indian Subcontinent

Ayurveda is the ancient alternative medicine of India going back about 5000 years; much of it essentially discredited today. In surgery, however, the Indian subcontinent was extremely advanced. Operative procedures included Cesarean sections and plastic surgery. Indian surgeons taught their Western contemporaries the art of rhinoplasty. The Hindu caste system, initiated in 1500 BC, distinguishes, in descending order, five primary categories: Brahims, Kshatriyas, Vaishyas, Shudras, and Dalits (the Untouchables). Healthcare statistically decreased as a descending function of caste, especially evident in the lack of healthcare for the Dalits. The healthcare underprivileged in India, in the past and in the present, includes hundreds of millions of people.

Ancient Greece

Although today's medicine had its origins in ancient Greece, the principles of Greek medical practice were suspended for nearly 2000 years. The foundation of ancient Greek medicine was the holistic concept of a healthy mind and a healthy body determined by internal humors or forces, today called metabolic processes. The medical practices of Asclepius and Hippocrates were focused on a scientific approach, the study of anatomy, the influence of environmental and psychological factors, as well as stressing the importance of the morality of the practitioner. The doctor/patient relationship emphasized maintaining confidentiality and trust. The democracy of Athens established a public health system of doctors elected by the populace for their merits, paid for by the state and obligated to treat citizens, residents, former slaves set free, and current slaves—essentially everyone. These doctors visited and treated poor patients for free. For those who could afford a private physician, the amount of payment was a uniform one drachma, or, at the discretion of the patient. Hippocrates advised physicians not to determine their payment in advance because this might hinder the patient from seeking therapy. In essence, ancient Greece practiced universal healthcare; the wealth or poverty of patients was officially not a factor. In theory and probably also in practice, there were no healthcare underprivileged in ancient Greece.

Ancient Rome

The civilization of Rome dominated the Western World until 476 AD. The Romans adopted the principles and practices of ancient Greek medicine, augmented by battlefield and gladiatorial surgical knowledge. They used opium and scopolamine to relieve pain and vinegar to clean wounds. The Romans were firm believers in public health and personal hygiene to prevent the spread of disease. They built public baths, hospitals, clean water aqueducts, and toilets using a sewage system. Yet, the poor (the plebeians) lived shorter and more disease-afflicted lives than the rich (the patricians). Healthcare was not universal nor was it equitable. The disabled were not only underprivileged in their healthcare but ridiculed and ostracized for physical or mental impairments. Rome was a harsh world with little practice of philanthropy (the love of humankind).

Early Europe

After Rome there were no significant advances in healthcare except for battlefield surgery for centuries; instead, there was regression to superstition, magic incantations, poor hygiene, and a lack of public health. A dominance of ignorance exemplified medicine for the privileged as well as the underprivileged. Notable individual exceptions who promoted knowledge were for the most part ignored, like Paracelsus (1493–1541), primarily responsible for the introduction of chemical pharmaceutical preparations; Francis Bacon (1561–1626), who originated the steps of the scientific method; and William Harvey (1578–1657), who demonstrated the circulation of blood.

Modern medicine as we know it did not emerge until the Industrial Revolution of the eighteenth century when the Western World rediscovered Hippocrates and his Greek colleagues. Their teachings had persisted in the Byzantine Empire to 1493 and in the Arab cultures, influenced by the Persian physician Avicenna of the eleventh century. The nineteenth, twentieth, and early twenty-first centuries have seen a virtual explosion of medical knowledge and therapy, including the cure of many diseases, as well as vital improvements in surgery. Yet, throughout Europe and the New World, these advantages were not available to everyone. The poor have always been disadvantaged, and the majority of the disadvantaged poor belonged to a variety of racial or cultural groups, as well as to the multitudes of the disabled.

The USA

Though many in the USA today speak of healthcare as a "right," in actuality, healthcare in the USA has always been a privilege. The US inhabitants denied the fundamental existent healthcare of their time have been the underprivileged. In colonial times, the underprivileged were the majority. In our own time, they have gradually become the minority, but they are still very much present in considerable numbers in our society. The healthcare underprivileged have been and are primarily represented by certain identifiable groups disadvantaged because of their ethnicity or a disability.

Colonial Times

Life was harsh in colonial times. There was little science and no accepted body of fundamental medical knowledge. Doctors were few and mostly trained in individual apprenticeships. There were no government regulations related to public health. Malaria, diphtheria, and yellow fever were prevalent and life expectancy was around 40 years.

When rudimentary medical care was available it was fairly limited to the privileged Caucasian minority who could afford it. Except for home remedies, prayer, and witchcraft, the American black slave population had no recourse to healthcare. Not only were they overworked, they lacked proper nutrition, lived in overcrowded conditions, and lacked access to fundamental hygiene and sanitation. Such deprivations promoted poor healthcare and led to brutely short lives. When a slave was sick only the most privileged were seen by a doctor or given any medication or treatment. Average life expectancy of slaves was half that of the white population—about 20 years.

The 1800s; the Civil War

There was no improvement in healthcare in the USA of 1800. The childhood diseases of measles, mumps, chickenpox, and whooping cough were routine. Diarrhea from many pathogens, including dysentery and typhoid were common, especially in the Southern states. During the Civil War, more soldiers died of disease than from battle on both sides. Wounded officers in the Civil War had a better survival rate than did enlisted personnel because they were usually treated in private homes, whereas enlisted men were crowded into field hospitals; there they died from contagious infections and diseases.

Conversely, as has been common to most wars, the Civil War ushered in progress in surgical techniques, nursing, and research. After the Civil War, there was a surge in the building of hospitals, in particular by the US army. In a manner of speaking, hospitalization was government-supported socialized medicine for a privileged cohort. The majority of the population experienced little positive healthcare change. On a positive note, in 1899, the expansion of the American Medical Association to include half of the nation's physicians was a major healthcare achievement that introduced medical treatment standards.

The 1900s

The twentieth century was a watershed time for healthcare, raising national standards of treatment. The healthcare privileged had become the majority and the underprivileged the minority.

President Theodore Roosevelt advocated for health insurance and better national healthcare stating, "No country could be strong whose people were sick and poor." The terrible working conditions of the early industrial revolution promoted the rise of labor unions that provided health insurance for their members. A national compulsory health insurance mandate, however, was vigorously opposed by the private insurers, the American Medical Association, as well as by the unions themselves fearing a loss of their power. During World War I, a facsimile of the Veteran's Administration was initiated as the War Risk Insurance Program.

After the "Great War," non-profit health insurers, such as Blue Cross/Blue Shield entered the marketplace. The Social Security Act of 1935, signed by President Franklin D. Roosevelt, provided the first public support for the retired, elderly, unemployed, and disabled. Henry Kaiser, an industrialist, started pre-paid healthcare for his employees, an example that initiated nationwide employer-sponsored health insurance after World War II. President Lyndon B. Johnson signed the Social Security Act of 1965, with its originator, former President Harry S. Truman, at his side; this legislation laid the groundwork for Medicare and Medicaid. Healthcare legislation of some sort was advocated by the Republican right under President Richard Nixon and by the Democratic left under President John F. Kennedy—both without success.

Thus, the American hodgepodge of health insurance and healthcare availability was maintained throughout the 1900s. The remarkable benefits of the twentieth century medicine and surgery were available to most but certainly not to all.

Early 2000s

Four landmark events marked healthcare and the status of the healthcare underprivileged in the early twenty-first century: President Barack Obama's 2010 Affordable Care Act (ACA), or Obamacare, that established an open marketplace in which insurance companies could not deny coverage based on pre-existing conditions, an opportunity open to American citizens earning less than 400% of the poverty level. The second landmark event was the failure by President Donald Trump to undo the ACA. The COVID-19 crisis has been the third, totally focusing attention on the need for national healthcare. The fourth is the ever-increasing advocacy by the healthcare underprivileged for recognition and equality of medical care.

The Status of the Underprivileged in Current US Healthcare

Most authorities list five healthcare vulnerable populations in the USA in 2022: the chronically ill and disabled, low-income and homeless individuals, certain geographic (primarily isolated, rural) communities, the LGBTQ populations, and the very young and the very old. Individuals in this group, as a function of wealth, can be healthcare privileged or underprivileged. Group classification more amenable to analysis and probably to rectification is that of racial and ethnic distinctions. Today's preeminently healthcare underprivileged groups are: Native Americans, African Americans, Hispanic Americans, Asian Americans, and disabled Americans, as well as discrimination by gender prevalent in all of the above groups.

Native Americans

Native Americans have been underprivileged from the beginning of American settlement from the East. European settlers took their lands, killed their animal food supply (e.g., the buffalo), incarcerated them on reservations, and limited their work and educational opportunities. The first American citizens were considered second-rate citizens.

Pre-COVID-19, average US life expectancy in 2018 was 79.11 years; 77.4 years for Native Americans. A recent study showed Native American life expectancy to be as low as 68 years, the lowest in the USA, ten years lower than Hispanics, 7.7 years lower than Caucasians, and 2.7 years lower than that of African Americans. In every category of healthcare statistics, Native Americans fall below the average United

States' Caucasian citizen's average. These statistics include mortality rate, potential years life loss, infant mortality, amenable mortality to healthcare, healthcare access and quality index, and healthcare availability. As causes of death and affliction, Native Americans are particularly prone to a variety of cancers, diabetes, and kidney failure.

The Indian Health Service is a federal government agency under the United States Department of Health and Human Services. Their mission is to raise the physical, mental, social, and spiritual health of American Indians and Alaska natives. Eligibility for benefits is based on membership in one of the 574 federally recognized Indian tribes, living in 326 Indian land areas (22%) and in the rest of the nation, a total of 6.8 million people. Medical services are available on Indian reservations and in designated clinics outside the reservations. Leadership in the Indian Health Service is provided by tribal-affiliated Native Americans. Services include direct patient care and the initiation of public health measures. The Service employs 15,000 workers consisting of Civil Service federal employees and United States Public Health Service Commissioned Officers, overseen by the Surgeon General. Their number includes physicians, nurses, dentists, pharmacists, dieticians, and veterinarians. They provide for medical and dental care, behavioral health and rehabilitation services, as well as research opportunities in medicine and environmental health and engineering. The Service, however, is extremely underfunded with per capita healthcare spending only one-third of that of the rest of the nation.

It is unclear today if the ultimate goal of raising the healthcare of the Native American population to that of a standard US norm will best be met by the separate but equal efforts of the Indian Health Service or by the assimilation of today's underprivileged Native Americans into the US mainstream of healthcare.

African Americans

As slaves, African Americans had little to no professional healthcare and lived in terrible public health conditions. Healthcare for African Americans has markedly improved, but they remain among the most healthcare underprivileged of US citizens. By 2020, the average life expectancy of African Americans was 71.8 years, compared to 78.7 years for the entire population and 77.6 years for Caucasians. In addition to racial discrimination, the lack of wealth is a primary factor. While there are extremely affluent African Americans, for example, Hollywood stars and professional athletes who can afford the best of healthcare, the African American community, as a whole, suffers from unemployment, discriminatory wages, and limited job opportunities, resulting in a lack of insurance coverage and other means of purchasing standard US healthcare. It is incumbent on a just nation to provide healthcare equality for those we have made healthcare underprivileged. Changing this situation is a necessary goal and a moral imperative.

Hispanic Americans

Hispanics, including native- and foreign-born, are the largest ethnic minority in the USA. They comprise approximately 55 million people or 18% of the nation's population. Though Hispanic Americans have higher life expectancy (81.9 years in 2018) than Caucasians (78.6 years in 2018), they are among the healthcare underprivileged.

Hispanics perform a disproportional number of unskilled, high-risk jobs contributing to a lower average income. In 2014, the median household income of Hispanics was $39,600, in comparison to non-Hispanic Whites of $60,300. In 2014, 23.6% of Hispanics lived below the poverty level, in comparison to 14.89% of the national population. Additionally, about 25% of Hispanics are uninsured (about 10% for non-Hispanics). Poor healthcare again is primarily associated with poverty.

In addition, Hispanics, as a group, exhibit high rates of disease risk factors—obesity, tobacco smoking, and alcohol use, the forerunners of diabetes, cardiovascular disease, cancer, and liver disease. In association with language difficulties and a reluctance to seek medical care, therapeutic care for Hispanics is often not only late but too late.

Asian Americans

Though the approximately 24 million (7.24% of the total US population) Asian Americans enjoy the longest life expectancy of US citizens, 86.3 years in 2014, and are well represented in many upper income positions, especially in higher education, they are also an underprivileged healthcare segment of our nation. Statistically, Asian Americans, especially Cambodians and Vietnamese, are less likely to have a personal doctor and less likely to have prophylactic assessments of blood pressure, cancer screening, and routine mammograms and pap smears. They have a higher prevalence of cancer (particularly breast cancer in Vietnamese women), chronic obstructive pulmonary disease, hepatitis B, tuberculosis, and liver disease.

Disabled Americans

The largest number of US citizens whose healthcare is underprivileged are the 54 million Americans with physical, developmental, and psychological disabilities.

The ancient Greeks were ambivalent in their treatment of the disabled. Some were welcomed and prized in society; there was a form of Medicaid for the disabled in ancient Athens; conversely, infanticide of the deformed at birth was a common practice, especially in ancient Sparta. The practices of ancient Rome were even more cruel towards the disabled. They threw deformed infants into the Tiber River to drown, and they mutilated children to increase their value as beggars. The disabled were afforded better treatment in ancient Egypt where they were provided with medical care, artificial limbs, and other facilitating devices. In ancient China they were often revered and considered holy "wizards."

Until the 1900s, western healthcare was a prolonged Dark Ages for the disabled. Asylums hid the disabled from public view. In the 1950s the disability advocacy groups began to have an impact. Slowly, ever so slowly, common conveniences, special facilities, and equality of medical care were made available by law for our citizens with disabilities (e.g., Americans with Disabilities Act).

Unfortunately, people with disabilities tend to have more health problems and thus a greater need for healthcare. Women with significant disabilities sign up for fewer routine mammograms and pap smears; the deaf have a more difficult time communicating their health needs; the motility-impaired have physical limitations in obtaining healthcare access; and, the blind have been documented as experiencing significant levels of obesity and its metabolic syndrome comorbidities.

Conditions that challenge the disabled community in addition to bias include poverty and race. Explicit and implicit bias toward the disabled is prevalent throughout the non-disabled community. This bias is, at times, even exhibited by the healthcare workers to whom the disabled turn for medical help, understanding, and empathy. There is no question that the poorest healthcare in any underprivileged group is dominant in the poorest members of the group; in the US today, healthcare remains a relative function of personal economic resources. Therefore, already underprivileged by being disabled, Native Americans and African Americans are the most healthcare deprived among the disabled.

Gender

Healthcare gender discrimination was common among providers in the past. Until quite recently, women were excluded from or biased against in becoming doctors or medical specialists in certain disciplines. The great anesthesiologist, Dr. Virginia Apgar, author of the infant Apgar Score, and one of my teachers, wanted to be a surgeon, but no surgical residency program would admit her. This gender discrimination was common until the end of the twentieth century. Today, women surgical trainees are essentially equal in number to men; women graduates from medical schools number over 50%. Women, however, especially within the previously discussed societal segments of the healthcare disadvantaged, are still lacking equality of care in comparison to men.

In today's emphasis on diversity and gender equity there is hope and increasing evidence to substantiate the belief that within all underprivileged groups, gender equity will be the first to be achieved.

All of Us Are Healthcare Underprivileged

Chapter 1 statistically documents that, by all commonly employed quantifiable indices of healthcare, the USA is inferior to essentially every "Western" country of Europe, as well as to Australia, New Zealand, and our neighbor, Canada. Despite that fact, we pay more for our healthcare than any country in the world. Economically and socially privileged Americans are able to obtain the best medical care and enjoy the latest benefits of therapy, innovation, and comfort. But healthcare for the average US citizen is far below that standard.

We must eliminate second class healthcare in all segments of our population. We must make healthcare a right for all, rather than a realm for profiteering. Just as we believe that no one is above the law in our land, no one should experience less than the best available healthcare our country can provide. If we take pride in being "first among nations," first in uniform healthcare should be our goal.

Conclusions

Historically, healthcare has been a privilege reserved for a minority, with a majority, by definition, being underprivileged. Today, in the USA, the majority are privileged to receive standard national healthcare, but there is still a sizable group of the underprivileged, usually a function of income and assets. The healthcare disadvantaged are prevalent in Native Americans, African Americans, Hispanic Americans, Asian Americans, the disabled, and, though improving, in being female. In addition, US national healthcare is underprivileged in comparison to a large number of the countries in the world. Our national goal and our moral priority must be to achieve equity of healthcare for all of our citizens, as well as for our country to achieve healthcare parity with nations that provide the best in healthcare.

Sources

About the Affordable Care Act 2010. https://www.hhs.gov/healthcare.
An overview of the Americans with disabilities act 1990. https://adata.org/factsheet/ADA-overview.
It's Harder for People Living in Poverty to Get Health Care. https://www.commonwealthfund.org/publications/podcast/2019/apr/its-harder-people-living-poverty-get-health-care.

Chapter 10
Public Health and Pandemics

Healthcare is vital to all of us some of the time, but public health is vital to all of us all of the time.

C. Everett Koop, U.S. Surgeon General

Very Short Stories

Sanskrit writings (15th BC) include instructions on boiling water to make it safe to drink.

Ancient Rome (800–734 BC) had flush waste latrines that created public health protection from enteric diseases; this innovation was subsequently abandoned for centuries.

Ignaz Semmelweis (1818–1875) and Joseph Lister (1826–1912) were, at first, ridiculed for researching and advocating the washing of hands by doctors; they were subsequently vindicated, and their work has saved millions of patient lives.

Ancel Keys (1904-2004), Henry Blackburn (1925–), Henry Taylor (1912–1983), Jeremiah Stamler (1919–), pioneers of preventative medicine and public health, demonstrated to the world that lowering cholesterol with the Mediterranean diet, controlling blood pressure, and stopping cigarette smoking, would cause a substantial decline in atherosclerotic cardiovascular disease.

The role of public health and the agencies responsible for their contributions are often not given the credit they deserve for increasing the health of individuals. Without the successes of the functions and activities of public health a sustainable society, a civilization, would not be feasible or lasting.

A primary task of public health is to prevent, if possible, halt when necessary, and irradicate if feasible, the cause of an epidemic or pandemic. In this regard, the first responders to our national COVID-19 healthcare crisis, the doctors, nurses, and staff of medical providers reacted most admirably, at the risk of their own lives, to save individuals and to serve the public health in attempting to stem the tide of this deadly disease. The difficulty of this task, however, is illustrated in this chapter in the history of epidemics and pandemics. So many lessons of past epidemics and

H. Buchwald, *Healthcare Upside Down*, https://doi.org/10.1007/978-3-031-07163-8_10

pandemics have not been learned. Knowledge of successful interventions from prior public health catastrophes, often attained at a deadly cost, have been ignored.

Except for the cited first responders and the rapid development of vaccines, the US public health response to COVID-19 was a failure (Chap. 11). There were multiple causes for this failure: the disjointed, unsubstantiated, inaccurate mandates, policies, and statements of our national, state, and local governments; the subjugating of ethics to fear of losing employment responsible for the erroneous, belated, and contradictory proclamations of our healthcare officials sworn to protect the lives and health of our nation; the ignoring and minimizing of science and statistically sound data; the attitude of a large segment of our population. All these elements were responsible for a lack of true public health community measures for COVID-19; their roots were already present in the culture discussed in prior chapters.

Public Health Definition

Public health is a science dedicated to protecting and improving the health of communities and their inhabitants by researching and advocating the prevention of disease and injury, promoting healthy lifestyles, and being continuously vigilant in detecting and responding to infectious diseases. For example, the public health advocacy of sanitation has done more for the healthcare of humanity than any drug, operation, or other therapeutic option. Providing safe drinking water, proper disposal of wastes, and cleanliness have allowed the populations of the world to grow, cities and countries to flourish, human life expectancy to increase, and daily living to be less hazardous.

United States Public Health Service and Its Performance

The United States Public Health Service is a division of the Department of Health and Human Services. The Service was formed in 1798 during the presidency of John Adams as a system of marine hospitals. It rapidly expanded and today its scope is gargantuan. The Service encompasses the National Institutes of Health (NIH), the Centers for Disease Control and Prevention (CDC), the Indian Health Service (IHS), the Food and Drug Administration (FDA), the Agency for Toxic Substances and Disease Registry (ATSDR), the Health Resources and Service Administration (HRSA), the Agency for Healthcare Research and Equality (AHRQ), the Substance Abuse and Mental Health Services Administration (SAMHSA), the Public Health Service Commissioned Corps (PHSCC) led by the Surgeon General, and several other agencies. This array of taxpayer-supported agencies, each separately and conjointly, is relied upon by the public to protect the health of the nation. Most of the $1.3 trillion annual budget of the Department of Health and Human Services goes to healthcare.

The United States Public Health Service has, on the whole, performed adequately but not outstandingly in their obligations to safeguard and improve the overall health of our citizens. Though outstanding healthcare is available to many, it may not be available to the poor in our society. For example, many communities in our country suffer from air and water pollution. The average quality of life provided by healthcare is not optimal. In prior chapters, I have offered examples of healthcare for the individual; healthcare for all is the dismal product. The comparison of US national with international healthcare statistics cited in Chap. 1 clearly documents that US public health is far from praiseworthy or even acceptable.

Public health officials can recommend public policies, and, rarely, even mandate them. Historically, scientifically sound public health recommendations have met with public acceptance; however, nearly every beneficial public health recommendation has been met with opposition and disobedience by a substantial segment of the population, at times including community leaders and members of the medical profession.

Rarely does history not repeat itself. The truth is evident in the story of vaccinations, starting with its origins—the overcoming of virulent opposition from a segment of the public and eventually becoming a public health legacy of success.

Smallpox is an old disease with visual evidence of its presence dating back to the mummy of Ramses V, who died in 1157 BC. Estimates are that 400,000 people died annually from smallpox in Europe in the eighteenth century and that 500 million died in the 100 years prior to its eradication. The death toll for the infected population was 30%. Yet it was halted and eliminated by 1980, when the World Health Organization (WHO) certified its global eradication. The cause of this unique victory over smallpox was vaccination.

Immunization against smallpox started with live smallpox virus in China in the tenth century AD. Lady Mary Wortley Montagu promoted the procedure in England in 1718. George Washington, who survived smallpox in his youth, in 1777, as Commander-in-Chief of the Continental Armies, ordered all the troops to be immunized. This variolation approach with a live virus, however, leads to active, contagious smallpox in a small minority of people treated, with a 0.5–2.0% mortality rate.

In 1796, Edward Jenner produced smallpox immunity with a cowpox preparation and coined the word "vaccination" from the word "Vacca," for cow. The source of vaccine became the *vaccinia* virus in the nineteenth century, a genetically distant relative of cowpox and the *variola* virus of smallpox. The vaccine was 95% effective, with an 0.1% incidence of non-life-threatening side effects and a fatal response of 0.000198%. Vaccination against smallpox spread rapidly and soon was made mandatory by many nations. Between 1843 and 1855, the individual states of the USA required smallpox vaccination for all of their citizens. Global vaccinations occurred everywhere, from East to West, South to North, in the rich and the poor, and all races, creeds, and religions. Through these means, herd immunity was facilitated, and as global immunity became universal, smallpox vaccinations were discontinued in the 1970s.

This success story for humankind was not achieved without opposition. In 1802, the British cartoonist James Killray published a depiction of cowpox vaccination showing cows immerging from different parts of young women's bodies. In the 1800s, there were anti-smallpox vaccination leagues in England and the USA. The arguments of justification for these anti-vaxxers, as well as other anti-vaxxers throughout history have all been quite similar; namely, the claims that vaccination infringed upon personal liberties and religious beliefs, conspiracy theories of various kinds, and political party motivations.

Whatever their reasoning, the anti-vaxxers, in addition to opposing the best recommendation of public health, are in fundamental opposition to the law and order necessary for a society to function. The basis of community law is to safeguard life and minimize risk for harm. Anti-vaxxers make a decision not only for themselves but for their neighbors, fellow citizens, and families; they violate the underpinning of public safety and basic societal responsibility. Ironically, their opposition bring disease, hospitalization, and death, most of all to fellow anti-vaccination advocates.

Public Health and Individual Health

Public health depends upon the medical knowledge of the past, works to benefit medicine in the present, and plans for the future of a nation's health. Indeed, the lives and health of all of civilization rest upon these contributions. In this regard, however, the recommendations of health workers and researchers can, at times, be at odds with the welfare of members of a community.

For the sake of the common good, a well-functioning public health system may be required to create restrictions that can negatively impact an individual's physical and mental health. For example, employing isolation, quarantining, and social distancing during an epidemic may have interfered with the ability of individuals to seek healthcare for essential medical problems, such as cancer and heart disease. In addition, pandemics cause major psychologic problems in the world's populations and documented increases in suicide rates.

The converse is also true: individual health concerns can run contrary to what is best for the public health. As a modern example, treating an accident or heart attack victim with COVID-19 with mouth-to-mouth resuscitation, rushing the patient to a hospital for immediate care, bringing the person into an emergency room, general hospital ward, or the operating room, can expose many individuals to COVID-19 transmission.

As I documented in prior chapters, the current status of healthcare in the USA falls short of our expectations. In a more perfect world, public health policies and institutions would benefit all individuals, and the health of every citizen would contribute to public health.

Epidemics and Pandemics

The greatest challenges to a public health system and to emerging research are epidemics and pandemics. Past plagues have been universal crises that should have taught us lessons for the future. Unfortunately, the lessons of the past have rarely been heeded.

There have been many notable, historic epidemics and pandemics, dating back to 3000 B.C., with the Hamin Mangha/Miazigau epidemic that, from evidence of mass burial sites, swept through China.

Starting about 2500 years ago, we have written records of mass human exterminations. These include:

The Plague of Athens, 430–425 B.C., caused 100,000 deaths, one-third of the city of Athens, and was probably caused by typhoid fever.

The Antonine Plague, 165–180 A.D., caused 5,000,000 deaths, decimated the Roman Legions; the agent was smallpox.

The Plague of Cyprian, 250–271 A.D., killed 5000 people a day at its peak out of a population of 1,000,000, contributed to the fall of the Roman Empire; the agent was a virus.

The Plague of Justinian, 541–542 A.D., with recurrences until 750 A.D., caused up to 1,000,000 deaths, contributed to the fall of the Byzantine Empire; the agent was the bubonic plague bacterium.

The Black Death, 1346–1353 A.D., caused up to 200,000,000 deaths in one-third to one-half of Europe and Eurasia; the agent was bubonic plague bacterium.

The Cocoliztli Epidemic, 1545–1548 A.D., caused 15,000,000 deaths; the agent was Salmonella bacterium.

The Russian Flu Pandemic, 1889–1890 A.D., caused 1,000,000 deaths; the agent was Influenza A virus.

The Spanish Flu, 1918–1920 A.D., caused 50,000,000 deaths; the agent was Influenza A virus.

The Avian Flu, 1956–1958 A.D., caused 2,000,000 deaths; the agent was Influenza A virus.

SARS, 2002–2004 A.D., caused 800 deaths of the 8000 infected; the agent was SARS-CoV virus.

MERS, 2009–2012 A.D., caused about 800 hundred deaths of the 2000 infected; the agent was MERS-CoV virus.

The Swine Flu Pandemic, 2009–2010 A.D., caused about 500,000 deaths; the agent was Influenza A virus.

The Ebola Epidemics, 2014–2020 A.D., caused about 11,000 deaths with a 50% mortality; the agent was Ebola viruses.

Lessons Learned

Certain public health information has been gained by studying these scourges: Epidemics and pandemics have been recurrent throughout history. Many are zoonotic in origin, emanating from wild host mammals. Deaths have usually been higher in older individuals and in those with chronic diseases. Crowding, travel, and commerce promote dissemination. Segments of afflicted populations have often blamed these plagues on other segments of the population, in particular minority religious groups.

Social distancing, isolation, and quarantine were introduced in the fourteenth century for disease containment. The "Plague Doctors" of the fourteenth century who tended to the sick and dying during the Black Death introduced masking. They wore characteristic face masks with a bird-like beak made of leather and eyepieces of glass, filled with scented herbs that acted as a filter against airborne spread of infection. Global containment measures, learned over the past thousands of years, were successfully employed to keep the SARS, MERS, and Ebola viruses out of the USA.

Methods for combating plagues—mandatory face masks, social distancing, isolation, and quarantine, as well as the concept of asymptomatic transmission, to prevent resurgence of disease were well established before COVID-19. These injunctions, however, were delayed, ignored, or dismissed when COVID-19 became manifest (Chap. 11).

Epidemics and pandemics eventually end or are suppressed for a period of time without intervention. They are checked by herd immunity when a sufficient number of the population have died or have had the disease, and the infectious agent cannot find a susceptible host. At times, a variant of the pandemic agent that does not attack humans is created by mutation and becomes dominant. Historically, before either of these pandemic endpoints have been reached, global genocide has occurred, and at times entire civilizations have been annihilated.

Conclusions

The public health sector of healthcare is responsible for the general health of a nation. Pandemics have killed and maimed more people than world wars and appear to be inevitable. The practices of public health are necessary to combat pandemics. Public health in the US was suboptimal prior to COVID-19, and, except for the rapid deployment of first responders and the development of vaccines, a societal failure during the COVID-19 pandemic.

Sources

Breen JJ. Pollution prevention in industrial processes. – ACS. Publication. 1992; https://bups.acs.org/doi/pdf
CDC. Water treatment/public water systems/drinking water. https://www.cdc.gov/healthywater.
Mara D, et al. Sanitation and health. https://doi.org/10.1371/journal.pmed.1000363.
U.S. Environmental Protection Agency. Wastes: what are the trends in wastes and their effects on human health and the environment? https://www.epa.gov/report-environment/wastes.

Chapter 11
COVID-19

We have it totally under control. It's one person coming in from China, and we have it under control. It's going to be just fine.

Donald Trump, Former U.S. President, January 22, 2020

This isn't a pandemic or just a virus. This is a pandemic of emotion. This is a pandemic of pain and suffering that has to do with lost jobs and lost persons… This is not a public health journey. This is really a personal journey for all of us.

Michael Osterholm, American Epidemiologist, March 23, 2021

A Story

Dr. Thomas Tuttle, born in Fulton, Missouri in 1869, was the Commissioner of Health for the State of Washington in 1918. The Spanish Flu of 1918–1920 came in three horrendous waves, the latter waves more deadly than the first. Five hundred million people were infected worldwide (28% of the world's population) and 50 million died (10% mortality). To combat this scourge, Dr. Tuttle made wearing face masks mandatory; he advocated social distancing; he encouraged home isolation and quarantining of individuals who had been exposed to the virus; he raised the notion of asymptomatic transmission; he warned of a resurgence of disease if restrictions were lifted too early. His efforts were met with great societal opposition. In response, the United States Public Health Service terminated Dr. Tuttle's appointment as Commissioner of Health and dismissed him from the Service.

To illustrate the fact that current healthcare in the USA is far from what it should be, every chapter has demonstrated the flaws in our current system. However, in the story of the US response to COVID-19, the greatest opportunity for redemption resided. The actions of the first responders to COVID-19, the doctors, nurses, ambulance attendants, and other healthcare workers, who at the risk of their own lives, provided acute care for the sick give us all hope for the future of healthcare. Yet, it is important to study the reality of the full US response to the COVID-19 pandemic, its fallacies and the lessons to be learned. The US response in confronting the COVID-19 pandemic provides a most devastating example of a nation's failure to

H. Buchwald, *Healthcare Upside Down*, https://doi.org/10.1007/978-3-031-07163-8_11

meet a healthcare crisis. Perhaps that failure to head off the American pandemic will engender national reflection and begin the process of true preparation for the future. Only healthcare reform will be an acceptable tribute to the COVID-19 dead, their grieving families, and all those who suffer and continue to suffer from this disease.

The Statistics

Table 11.1 displays the discouraging COVID-19 pandemic statistics for the world, the USA, and comparable data for several other countries through March 2021. Though the world pandemic data continuously evolved, this dataset represents the outcomes of the beginning year or so of the pandemic.

With about 4.3% of the world's population, the USA had 25.1% of the number of recorded cases, as well as 20.1% of the world's deaths and 482% (1585 US/326.8 world) of world deaths per one million citizens.

The countries ranked one to five in COVID-19 deaths and recorded cases were: USA, India, Brazil, Russia, UK. In none of the four nations ranked below the USA did the COVID-19 death rate reach one-half of that in the USA, and the total number of cases in any of these nations was less than 38% of that of the USA. Only in deaths per million population was the USA exceeded by any nation, namely the UK.

In stark contrast, China where the COVID-19 pandemic started was ranked 85, with a population about four times that of the USA, and total reported deaths of 4636, which is less than 1% of that of the USA, and only three deaths per million, which is less than 0.2% that of the USA. Of course, we do not know if that data can be trusted. Subsequently, China experienced a huge surge in the number of cases and in districts afflicted.

A country whose data we can trust as truly factual is New Zealand. This nation of approximately five million people was ranked 174 and by March of 2021 had only 2378 total cases, with 26 deaths, five per million. Correcting for population size, the incidence of cases in New Zealand in comparison to the USA was 0.008%, the number of deaths less than 0.005%, and the deaths per million population 0.32%. Unfortunately, as the world scourge of COVID-19 surged fairly unabated, the early

Table 11.1 COVID-19 data March 2021

Country	Population	Deaths	Deaths/million	Total infections
World	7,674,532,974	2,547,376	326.8	114,932,072
1. USA	332,288,557	526,838	1585	29,292,589
2. India	1,388,575,299	157,257	113	11,222,986
3. Brazil	213,559,824	255,018	1197	10,551,259
4. Russia	145,376,545	86,455	592	4,257,650
5. UK	68,122,332	122,953	1805	4,182,009
85. China	1,439,323,776	4636	3	89,912
174. New Zealand	5,002,100	26	5	2378

New Zealand triumph diminished; however, New Zealand maintained superiority in COVID-19 disease control in comparison to the USA.

The USA, therefore, in the incidence and fatalities of COVID-19 after the first year of the pandemic was first in the world by very wide margins. By June of 2021, the average US life expectancy, as a direct consequence of the COVID-19 pandemic, had plummeted 1.9 years, 8.5-fold that of any other developed nation.

Responsibility

As a nation, we responded too late, inappropriately, and disjointedly. The statistics do not lie; neither do the documented actions or lack of actions, by government, healthcare agencies and resources, and segments of the public.

Government

The federal government closed the gateways into our country in inadequate stages and only after the COVID-19 virus was already well established in the USA. The federal government minimized and continued to minimize the impact of the pandemic, even in the face of horrendous death rates in Europe and within the USA. The federal government was extremely late in recruiting pharmaceutical companies to manufacture sufficient quantities of vaccine and to discover an appropriate therapeutic or preventative anti-viral drug. Above all, the federal government failed to support nationwide centuries-proven, effective means to limit viral exposure by masking, social distancing, hand washing, and closing or limiting establishments of community congregation. The advocacy of these simple public health measures was met by the federal government with disdain, ridicule, and, at times, punishment for its advocates.

Each state government inaugurated its own COVID-19 response. Some states attempted to reduce viral exposure by closing schools, restaurants, bars, and limiting gatherings in houses of worship. Other states practiced business as usual, as if this scourge was not sweeping through cities and countryside, a miasma carrying grave illness and death. The mayors of cities and governing councils throughout the country displayed ambivalence and confusion.

Overall, the response of government officials appeared to be guided by considerations of re-election rather than by following appropriate public health measures.

The Public

The public response during 2020, the year of confusion, was mixed. Many older people, the most COVID-19 vulnerable, practiced isolation. Travel sharply decreased and travelers sustained periods of quarantine. Certain public businesses voluntarily restricted customer exposure or closed their doors, and people not influenced by inaccurate information wore masks outside of the home, eliminated or reduced family get-togethers, practiced social distancing, and waited for the availability of national vaccination.

There were many citizens, however, who refused to practice any of these prophylactic measures, claiming that they violated their rights as citizens, their freedom of choice, or their personal or religious beliefs. Though in the USA, we hold individual choice as sacred, should that choice be sanctioned if it endangers the lives of others? For example, not masking is a choice a person can make for her/his own safety, but not masking clearly indicates that the individual does not care about exposing others to the virus and, possibly, as a result, killing others.

The Economy

Often in the national debate of what should be or should not be done to limit COVID-19, the issue of the economy was raised. There is no question that many businesses suffered; as in every national crisis, some prospered. It is ironic that the annual incomes of some healthcare institutions and that of their CEOs actually rose during the pandemic, at the expense of the suffering public. Incomes of US CEOs overall rose 5% in 2020 from their 2019 levels for a median income of $12.7 million as 61% of CEOs saw an increase in their take-home dollars in 2020.

Essentially every economist will tell you that prolongation of a pandemic will be more economically damaging than short-term sacrifices, thereby justifying anti-pandemic government spending. The US government stimulus payments to nearly every household in part offset the deprivations of COVID-19, including the profiteering by healthcare insurers, some of whom refused to pay for certain COVID-19 medical expenses.

Healthcare Agencies and Experts

Major responsibility for our healthcare response to COVID-19 must be borne by our public health institutions and officials. Their actions can be summarized simply as too little, too late, and inappropriate.

The Centers for Disease Control and Prevention (CDC) is a national public health institution under the Department of Health and Human Services, whose mission is defined as: "To promote health and quality of life by preventing and controlling disease, injury, and disability." To facilitate this task, the CDC has an annual budget of about $160 million. Robert R. Redfield, a virologist, was CDC Director in 2020. In February 2020, the CDC's early COVID-19 test malfunctioned nationwide due to violation of its own protocols; in March 2020, Dr. Redfield told Congress that the COVID-19 testing system was "not geared to what we need right now." Only in

July 2020, 6 months after COVID-19 had entered and run rampant in the USA, did Redfield call for the wearing of masks. Throughout the pandemic, the CDC never issued a scientific assessment of the range of masks advocated and employed. In July 2020, the CDC proposed the reopening of schools even though its own data showed an acceleration of the US pandemic. Redfield resigned in January 2021.

The COVID-19 response of the National Institutes of Health (NIH) was predominantly represented by the public pronouncements of Dr. Anthony S. Fauci, Director of the National Institute of Allergy and Infectious Diseases (NIAID) and advisor to six US presidents. His statements were eminently sound but often contradicted by President Trump.

The Surgeon General of the United States is the operational head of the U.S. Public Health Services Commissioned Corps and the leading designated spokesperson on matters of public health in the federal government. The Surgeon General for the COVID-19 crisis year 2020 was Vice Admiral Jerome Adams. In the beginning of our national COVID-19 epidemic, Adams aligned himself with President Trump and downplayed the risk of COVID-19 by comparing it to the seasonal flu. Early in the pandemic he implored people not to buy or use face masks in public stating that they were ineffective. Dr. Adams was asked by President Biden to step down as Surgeon General in January 2021.

The first COVID-19 vaccine became available in the USA in December of 2020 and proved to be 95% effective against the then current COVID-19 variant. The US regulators of the Food and Drug Administration (FDA) only gave full approval of its use in August of 2021, over 8 months later. This delay prevented the vaccination of a vast number of Americans before the full-strength arrival of the delta variant, encouraged anti-vaccinators, and prevented government institutions, including universities and the military, from mandating vaccination. Why did the FDA do this? It is difficult to find a scientific reason for this major policy decision; as a political decision, it is frightening.

What Is SARS-COV-2, the Cause of COVID-19?

A virus is distinguished from a bacterium by its microscopic size and in being unable to replicate itself outside of a host cell. The SARS-CoV-2 that causes COVID-19 consists of a single-strain of a ribonucleic acid (RNA) chemical that carries the formula for its genetic structure. Bound to this RNA string are nucleoproteins that give the virus its spatial structure. Encapsulating this viral core is a lipid envelope with protruding spike proteins. These spike proteins allow the virus to penetrate a host cell. Once inside the cell, the virus instructs the mitochondria, the production factory of the cell, to make more of itself, until the virus-saturated cell ruptures, spreading the newly formed viral progeny.

The virus of COVID-19 is a chemical, not an intellectual entity, obeying its programmed instructions for its survival. Humans are an essential source for its perpetuation; in serving that purpose all humans are equally at risk from the virus. A chemical does not favor the policies of a political party or politician. A chemical is entirely unaware of the complex beliefs of religion, laws, national constitutions. Yet, every day, this particular chemical promotes misery, kills, and destroys the structure of our society. Though it is the enemy of all of us, it is still only a chemical without a creed.

Beating COVID-19

Societal Isolation

The universal adherence to wearing masks, social distancing, washing hands, restricting group travel, avoiding large gatherings, and judicious access to schools and other facilities is highly successful in limiting infection and even in eliminating infection.

Vaccines

Effective vaccination of most of a country's citizens is, of course, the best way to eliminate COVID-19. Even if vaccines provide limited protection but minimize the symptoms and prevent death, they are valuable and will contribute to herd immunity. The future will determine if booster shots of a vaccine are effective and needed. If virus variants resist the early vaccines, vaccination adjustments may be sufficient to restore desired immunity.

Drugs

Effective oral pharmaceuticals can be developed to treat COVID-19 infections, comparable to taking penicillin for a strep throat. The same agents, or others, taken daily, can be useful in preventing COVID-19. Intravenous or subcutaneous COVID-19 antibodies can be used to treat early disease or given prophylactically to individuals with primary (congenital) or secondary (transplant patients) immunodeficiency syndromes.

Nature

Before vaccines and before drugs, major pandemics came and went. If the infectious agent is not able to find human access due to herd immunity or because a dominant mutant variant loses virulence, the pandemic, rather than its victims, will die out.

First Responders

Excellent healthcare, national preparedness, and community unity can prevent future pandemics or rapidly bring them under control. Ebola epidemics have devastated parts of Equatorial Africa, but only four cases of Ebola virus disease occurred in the USA and the disease never spread beyond hospital containment. With realistic government guidance, and the appropriate function of our healthcare institutions, we might similarly have been able to avoid the deadly consequences of COVID-19 in the USA.

Conclusions

We could have done better with our national response to COVID-19. We could have made use of the lessons learned from previous pandemics (Chap. 9). Though our first responders performed admirably, public support came only from part of the populace. Government policies were irresponsible. Our healthcare agencies and experts were derelict in their sworn duty to protect the public. In the future, our country must separate science from politics in healthcare.

Sources

CDC Coronavirus Disease (COVID-19). https://www.cdc.gov/covid
COVID Live - Coronavirus Statistics - Worldometer. https://www.worldometers.info
Osterholm MT, Emanuel E. The omicron surge could be the worst public health challenge of our lifetime. Dec 30, 2021. https://www.washingtonpost.com/opinions/2021/12/30/omicron-variant-challenges-covid/.
Wang C, et al. Comparative study of government response measures and epidemic trends for COVID-19 global pandemic. Risk Anal. 2022;42(1):40–55. https://doi.org/10.1111/risa.13817.
World Health Organization: WHO Coronavirus (COVID-19) Dashboard. https://covid19.who.int/.

Chapter 12
Research

In the lively leavens of an atmosphere fostering inquiry, no one
was afraid to come forward with a novel idea, no matter how
strange or unfamiliar it may have sounded. The stages of a new
idea are multiple. Many are stillborn. But every new suggestion
deserves at least a trial of being blown upon in the hope that
there may be sparks in the ashes.

Owen H. Wangensteen, Journal of the American Medical
Association, 1968

The true sign of intelligence is not knowledge but imagination.

Albert Einstein, Scientist

A Short True Story

After years of careful laboratory research, on March 26, 1954, a one-year-old boy
was rolled into the operating room at the University of Minnesota. Cross-circulation
of blood with his father, acting as a heart-lung machine, was established. The boy's
chest and then heart were opened by Drs. C. Walton Lillehei and Richard L. Varco.
As expected, a ventricular septal defect, a hole between the right and left ventricles
of the heart was visualized. Dr. Lillehei sewed it shut. The baby's heart and chest
were closed, and he was removed from cross-circulation. The operation was a success; however, the boy's heart failure had progressed beyond repair, and he died.
The next two children with a ventricular septal defect operated on by Dr. Lillehei
and his team by cross-circulation lived. In 1955, Dr. Richard DeWall's bubble oxy-
genator was introduced to replace cross-circulation. Open heart surgery was on its
way. Millions of children with congenital heart defects subsequently benefitted
from these initial efforts. Open heart surgery for a great variety of problems is now
routine in most of the world.

There are several lessons in this story; most important is that research has been
the predecessor of progress in healthcare and that without scientific research the
world would be a far poorer place inhabited by disease, congenital anomalies, and
death. Any progress in the healthcare statistics enumerated in Chap. 1 started with

research by an individual, a group, or an institution. At times, research involves failure; to overcome failure requires perseverance, as well as faith in sound convictions, always keeping sight of the ultimate goal of alleviating suffering and promoting life.

Definition and Origin of Research

Research is the systematic investigation of a prior or current belief or practice to ascertain its validity and to illuminate a path or paths to progress. In eras without research, civilization stood still, frozen in time. Western history has had those static eras when there was little research, e.g., the Dark Ages between the decline of the dynamic Roman Empire endowed with the lessons of the Classic Period and the explosive Renaissance age with its pursuit of knowledge. In those years of tumultuous change, research thrived in the arts, in government, in health, in travel, in the comforts of living, and, of course, in warfare.

Experimentation, the basis of research, dates back to the earliest thinking about cause and mechanisms. Research was championed by the Greek philosopher Aristotle. His predecessor, Hippocrates, known as the father of medicine, endorsed healthcare premises based on his experimental studies that are relevant today. In Renaissance England, Sir Francis Bacon, 1561–1626, is credited with defining the step-wise scientific method of: observation of phenomena, questioning of assumptions, formulation of a hypothesis, testing the hypothesis, converting a validated hypothesis to a theory, testing the theory by a trial, the derivation of conclusions, and establishing confirmed facts.

Research and Pandemics

Research utilizing the scientific method has made major contributions in understanding and stopping pandemics. Variolation, the injection of a small quantity of a live virus, for smallpox was introduced from Africa to Europe and the Americas in 1720. Jenner, in 1796, initiated vaccination, the injection of an attenuated virus, using the cowpox virus, which offered protection against the variola virus of smallpox. The first flu virus vaccines were developed in the 1930s, with large scale availability beginning in 1945. A vaccine against the Ebola virus was developed in 2016. In record time, multiple COVID-19 vaccines were created in the winter of 2020–2021. However, a multipotential anti-viral vaccine, applicable to several species of virus and their variants has yet to become a reality. Ongoing research to develop vaccines against pandemic pathogens is the strongest defense against future pandemics.

The quest for anti-viral pharmaceuticals has not been as successful as the field of antibiotics for bacterial diseases, in part, due to greater species variability and rapidity of mutations. Anti-viral drugs were not produced until the 1950s; one of the earliest available was methisazone used against smallpox in the 1960s. It would be an outstanding victory to cure, rather than only to mitigate, active COVID-19 with a pill, as well as to be able to protect against acquiring COVID-19 with a prophylactic medication comparable to the agents available to prevent malaria. Adequate funding to develop COVID-19 pharmaceuticals was not initiated until 2021, two years after the onset of the COVID-19 pandemic and after 500,000 US deaths. Before COVID-19, the economic perspective of drug companies deemed preparatory pandemic research to find anti-virals for pandemic containment not profitable enough to warrant substantial research funding.

Learning Research

Some researchers are self-taught, but most have some education in the rudiments of performing research in their schooling or in the academic, public health, and industry apprenticeships of today. The vast amount of scientific literature, available online, the huge existent databases, and the availability of electronic search engines have provided researchers with resources never dreamed of in generations past. For most, the availability of these facilities has offered great advantages; for others, however, they have been a detriment by extinguishing individual enthusiasm and belief in original thinking.

The best way to learn to do research is by doing it, preferably in the laboratory, clinic, or environment of an established investigator who is guide and mentor. Learning basic methodology for the work of a functioning laboratory is the first step; it avoids time spent repeating past errors and provides the novice researcher facility with the necessary and available technology of his/her chosen vocation.

As in most educational endeavors, research includes a stepwise process of progressive research learning. First, the novice works on a project of his/her mentor's, becoming a contributor and a co-worker. Next, the novice is given or asked to work on an original project under the guidance of the mentor. After a period of months or years, the novice is on his/her own—an investigator. All researchers do not become independent investigators; the majority prefer to be co-workers. This decision is a matter of self-knowledge and is not choosing a lesser role. Indeed, some of the most valuable contributions to science and healthcare have come from the efforts of multiple co-workers.

Medical schools and post-doctoral residencies and fellowship programs are the primary institutions for teaching research fundamentals. Certain medical schools provide didactic classes on research methodology and offer research laboratory electives. In some post-doctoral programs, time in the laboratory is offered but only rarely made mandatory. In Minnesota, in the Wangensteen era of 1930–1967, surgical residency training required a minimum of two years of basic laboratory research and a return to the classroom for a PhD degree. Those were the years of a surgical renaissance in the heartland by a Department of Surgery that in a thirty-plus year period revolutionized intestinal surgery for bowel obstruction; introduced modern open heart surgery and heart transplantation; initiated metabolic/bariatric surgery for obesity and its comorbidities; originated the partial ileal bypass operation to treat high cholesterol levels, the intervention modality for the first clinical trial to demonstrate the benefits of cholesterol lowering; and was the first in a number of other areas of innovation and progress in healthcare.

Research is also taught in privately funded research institutions and in industry, usually within a specific focus of investigation. There are apocryphal but true stories of great inventions originating in the garages of independent researchers, e.g., the cardiac pacemaker by Earl Bakken, founder of Medtronics.

A cardinal subject for researchers to understand is statistics—the intellectualization of probability. Be it for laboratory bench research, clinical investigation, the analysis of "big" computer data, or public health knowledge, the principles, techniques, and interpretation of data by statistical analysis are integral to research. A fundamental understanding of the meaning of the common convention of defining statistical significance as events occurring less than five times out of 100 is important in interpreting scientific data.

Funding Research

Research requires money to provide the researcher and laboratory staff with income, equipment, often expensive, and supplies, as well as ancillary costs for travel to scientific meetings and publication of results. These funds are derived from a variety of sources: The primary source is government, through the National Institutes of Health with a current annual budget of $39 billion, and other government agencies. These funds are, in essence, funds obtained from all of us by taxation. Funds from industry are derived from products paid for by all of us. And philanthropic foundations, groups, and individual's monies are also obtained from all of us from the fruits of private enterprise. In essence, we, the public, in one way or another, pay for healthcare research.

The Soul of Research

History has shown us that for research and its benefits to thrive, especially in the field of healthcare, research must be independent, unfettered, granted freedom of thought and action within the boundaries of ethical responsibility, as well as honestly and generously funded. Science does not flourish under the jurisdiction of an autocratic institution.

Einstein's quote in the beginning of this chapter tells us that research is an adventure, an exploration of the unknown. The researcher stands before the gates of knowledge and must choose a path to follow. If the researcher meets with failure, he/she needs to be prepared to start down a different road of inquiry. The researcher must also be able to recognize that an unexpected discovery may be more valuable than the results being sought. Fleming left his Petri dishes growing bacteria uncovered and was absent from his laboratory for a few days; a mold blew in the open window, settled on the bacteria, and killed them. On returning to his laboratory, Fleming could have thrown out his spoiled bacterial cultures as an end to the misadventure; instead, his mind was open to what he observed—he had discovered penicillin. Serendipity can be destiny.

Healthcare Research Upside Down

In the past, researchers hired by industry, by a private disease-focused research institution, or by academia funded by an industry or private institute grant, were provided a salary and benefits, as well as laboratory funds to work toward a specific goal or product. The medical school academic who chose to be a researcher needed to compete for and obtain a grant given to his/her institution, which controlled the distribution of funds. Independent academic clinician/researchers, in particular surgeons such as Drs. C. Walton Lillehei and Richard L. Varco whose research pioneered open heart surgery, paid part of their own personal income from their surgical earnings and certain of their research expenses, as well as contributing funds to the department of surgery and the university administration. Most university and departmental administrative support was primarily funded by a reasonable overhead allotment paid by the sources of the research funding.

With the vast twenty-first century expansion of administrative personnel and their assumption of total authority over the various aspects of healthcare, discussed in these chapters, all of the above research norms radically changed. The administocracy of universities, hospitals, healthcare conglomerates, and private healthcare institutions joined the ranks of the pharmaceutical and medical instrument companies in providing, first and foremost, for their own welfare with large incomes and privileges, derived from the labor of the actual healthcare workers and the deprivation of services from healthcare recipients. The primary concern of administocracy, in addition to retaining control, is increasing their ranks. The sheer number of administrators expanded exponentially resulting in the creation of multiple vice presidents, associates, and assistants. This administrative expansion required money.

In order to fund the expanding administocracy, clinicians are urged, indeed compelled, to spend most, if not all, of their working hours, in performing patient care, with no time left for research. Because most physicians have now become employees of the administration, they have little choice but to comply. Those most affected are surgical researchers, the potential Lilleheis and Varcos of today and tomorrow. Because they earn more in the operating room than in the laboratory, they are urged to operate rather than to perform research.

Administration also pirates funds from the overhead paid to an academic institution ostensibly in support of the funded research. The overhead percentage demanded by administration from non-NIH funders is negotiated but is often outrageous, and the amount the NIH must pay in overhead is a staggering 55% (more than double the percent of overhead paid twenty years ago). Thus, when the NIH awards a research grant to an academic institution in the amount of a million dollars in direct costs, including the investigator's salary, the salaries of laboratory personnel, equipment, supplies, and travel, the NIH must also pay an additional $550,000 to the university in overhead, not a penny of which goes to the enumerated direct expenses for the funded research. How many light bulbs and other minor facility needs require such an extravagant overhead percentage? In actuality, to a large extent, these monies go to the personal income and expenses of the administrators and the upkeep of their vast percent of university space. By paying such a huge overhead percentage, the funds available for direct research costs of the total allocated research budget are diminished. The monies of the NIH come from taxes. Who pays those taxes? You and me. Thus, for every two dollars the public coffers pay for research, more than an additional dollar is paid for the burgeoning expenses of the ruling healthcare administocracy.

Why is today's healthcare research upside down? If the time, independence, and dedication of the researcher are negated, the funding of research limited or spent wastefully, and the concept of research unappreciated, then healthcare research is minimized and denied its proper function to provide for healthcare progress and a future free of pandemics, with less disease, and longer, happier lives for all citizens.

Conclusions

Healthcare without research is stagnation; healthcare research is the pathway to healthcare progress. Today, research, in particular independent research, is curtailed and no longer cost-effective.

Sources

Armitage P, et al. Statistical methods in medical research. 4th ed. Hoboken: Wiley-Blackwell; 2002. https://doi.org/10.1002/9780470773666.
Brittannica. Scientific methods/definitions, steps, & application. https://www.britannica.com/science/scientific-method
Fletcher RH, Fletcher SW. Evidence-based approach to the medical literature. J Gen Intern Med. 1997;12(2):5–14. https://doi.org/10.1046/j.1525-1497.
National Institutes of Health (NIH). https://www.nih.gov/.

Chapter 13
Doctor/Patient Relationship

The good physician treats the disease; the great physician treats the patient who has the disease.

William Osler, Canadian/American Physician

A Story

Two friends (A and B) are talking:

A: I'm sad today.

B: Why?

A: I just learned that my doctor passed away.

B: Since when did you have a doctor?

A: A long time ago, I had my own doctor. He retired five years ago. Before then, he was my doctor for at least twenty years.

B: How did you find him?

A: When we first moved into town, I asked around for a good doctor. Several people said, "Dr. Jones is great." I made an appointment to see him together with my wife, and he agreed to be our family doctor.

B: I remember your wife's hip surgery and your heart attack. Did he take care of you for those problems?

A: He made all the arrangements for my wife's surgery, and he came to see her every day she was in the hospital. Then he chose a physical therapist. By the way, he picked the orthopedic surgeon, who is a lot like my doctor. She explained the surgery to us before she went into the operating room. She saw us before and after the operation, took care of my wife in the hospital, and continued to follow her for some time thereafter. Same with my heart attack. My doctor rushed me to the hospital and got a terrific cardiologist to treat me. The two of them pulled me through. I continue to see the cardiologist. When my doctor retired, I stayed with his clinic, but it had changed. I no longer had a doctor; I had a whole bunch, but none of them really seemed to care about me personally.

B: I know how you feel.

H. Buchwald, *Healthcare Upside Down*,
https://doi.org/10.1007/978-3-031-07163-8_13

Another Story
Two doctors (C and D) are talking:

C: Long day, fifteen minutes by the clock to see each patient. I have no idea how many patients I saw. The nurses do most of the hands-on work; the scribe makes the notes; I rarely see any patient twice.

D: That's what the electronic record system is for.

Both: (laugh)

C: You're a surgeon. Is your day more interesting?

D: I love being in the operating room, but I don't like being part of a service line team. Basically, I'm the technician who brings in most of the money for the group, and they take care of the patients and have the relationship. I remember the way it used to be. Today, I received a reminder from the past. I got a letter from a patient I took care of years ago, telling me about her life now, her job, her family. She thanked me for saving her life. I've received several such letters in the past, and I save them all; they keep me going. They remind me that once I was not only a technician but a doctor.

The Doctor/Patient Relationship

History

Most elements in our current civilization were foreshadowed in Ancient Egypt, from 4000–1000 BC. The doctors of that time were court dignitaries and priests. The physician Imhotep, 2650–2600 BC, was deified 2000 years after his death; Hesy-Ra, lived around 2670 BC, was known for his dentistry; Peseshet, who lived about 2500 BC, was stated to be a woman physician. These doctors prescribed medicines, performed surgery (e.g., circumcisions, setting of fractures, etc.), and offered prayers. Their relationship with their patients was determined by their hierarchical station—dominant to most, subservient to those of higher rank.

The Golden Age of Greek and Roman medicine, 500 BC to 476 AD, abandoned magical and religious justifications for human functions and introduced observation and experimentation. The practice of medicine moved somewhat closer toward being available to the average person. The cardinal contribution of that period in terms of the doctor/patient relationship was the often-quoted Hippocratic Oath, which established a mutual code of conduct for the physician and the patient: ...*into whatsoever houses I enter, I will enter to help the sick... And whatsoever I shall see or hear in the course of my profession, as well as outside my profession in my intercourse with men, if it be what should not be published abroad, I will never divulge, holding such things to be holy secrets....* These words established the patient's trust in the physician and the principle of doctor/patient confidentiality.

Once again superstition and religion dominated medicine in the Western World until the eighteenth century. They were minimized with the introduction of the precepts of liberalism and equality, wherein beliefs without evidence and autocratic prescriptions of remedies had no place. Early in the 1700s, symptoms were considered to be the illness and the defective organ was the problem. The doctor treated the patient's description of what ailed him or her. Later in that century, this emphasis was changed when doctors recognized that the symptoms were insights into the pathology. The physician, thereby, took charge of analysis, diagnosis, and therapy. The role of the "good patient" was to accept a passive role.

With the advent of psychology and its emphasis on perception and emotions, more attention in the doctor/patient relationship was focused on the patient as a unique entity. By the twentieth century, the concept of physician fallibility became more widespread and gained prominence by the acceleration of malpractice lawsuits in the 1960s. The response of practitioners, emphasized in the teachings of medical schools, was to establish a relationship of confidence with their patients based on transparency rather than declarations of authority.

Doctors learned to say, "let's try this," rather than, "do this;" and doctors were actually heard to say, "I don't know." Above all, mutual and independent satisfaction in the doctor/patient relationship was based on trust and the continuity of care that comes with trust. The doctor and the patient came to know each other, both aware that the doctor might not always be right but was trying his/her best, and that their relationship was based on honesty.

This relationship was taught at the root of the practice of medicine—in the medical schools of the past. Two concepts were emphasized: humanism and professionalism. Humanism prescribes that healthcare should be administered with honesty, empathy, compassion, altruism, and respect for the dignity and beliefs of patients and their families. Professionalism is manifested by values, behaviors, and relationships that underpin the trust the public has in its doctors. The relationship between doctor and patient is a social contract, a commitment to competence, integrity, and morality. In essence, these precepts are the modern expression of the Hippocratic Oath.

The concepts of obligation and responsibility have been codified, again and again, by professional representative bodies (e.g., the American Medical Association, the American College of Surgeons). These embodiments of principles and relationships in written codes of conduct serve as mandates for the practice of medicine.

Deterioration of the Doctor/Patient Relationship

In the twenty-first century, there is overwhelming evidence of the deterioration and actual disintegration of the doctor/patient relationship, which was based on the continuity of care that fosters trust, honesty, transparency, and respect. Many of today's doctors no longer assume the personal responsibility inherent in stating the words, "My patient;" and the patient no longer has the evidence to speak of, "My doctor."

In Chap. 1, I provided solid statistics demonstrating that the USA is markedly inferior to comparable nations in all major determinants of healthcare, except one, the cost of healthcare, in which the USA substantially leads all competitive nations.

In Chap. 2, I showed that language, the transformative precursor of reality, has depersonalized US healthcare and denigrated the integrity of the time-honored doctor/patient relationship. The patient has become "the client" and is a paying customer of a business primarily concerned with profits. The doctor is known as the "provider/employee," a service attendant for each of the client's visits to the healthcare business "firm." Different providers may see the client at each visit.

In Chaps. 3, 4, 5, and 6, I illustrated the dissolution of the doctor/patient relationship in medical schools, in patient clinics, in hospitals, and in the practice of US medicine today. In Chap. 7, I showed that a very few highly paid individuals profit from the current system and that their profit comes at the expense of both doctors and patients. In Chap. 8, I noted that socialized medicine is present in over 60% of US healthcare today, and that it is based on the loss of independence by both doctor and patient. In Chap. 9, I discussed the additional disadvantages faced by the underprivileged. In Chap. 10, I discussed the prescribed roles of our vast public health systems. In Chap. 11, I outlined the greatest failure of US healthcare, the COVID-19 pandemic. Part of the responsibility for the COVID-19 catastrophe was that certain doctors and healthcare leaders did not do their duty, and that some patients acted against their own best interests. A doctor/patient relationship based on mutual trust, assumption of responsibility, and respect for scientific principles might have helped to avoid a major part of the deaths and suffering of COVID-19. And, in Chap. 12, I discussed the role of research in assuring the future of healthcare administered by doctors to their patients.

Personal Recollections

I became a physician and practiced surgery well before the deterioration of the doctor/patient relationship. I have many illustrative personal recollections of how this association worked in the past and what it has come to be.

In Chap. 6, I related the evening visit of one of my medical school professors, who, on his own initiative, came to care for my wife who had the flu. When I left the post of Flight Surgeon, Strategic Air Command (SAC), US Air Force to start my surgical residency training, SAC placed me on immediate recall status until age forty and required me to have an annual flight status physical. I befriended a cardiologist in my new institution, who agreed to be my general physician and perform these examinations. He remained my doctor until his retirement, and we remained friends until he died in his mid-nineties.

Similarly, my wife had long-standing relationships with physicians and obstetricians, and our children were seen by a single pediatrician until they reached adulthood. Until the decline in the doctor/patient relationship, we visited "our" doctors for annual physicals, called them when ill, and trusted them for specialist referrals. All doctors readily responded to a telephone call.

Gradually, insidiously, this congenial, reliable, and reassuring availability of healthcare changed for my family. My status as Professor of Surgery at the University of Minnesota provided us with an advantage in obtaining excellent medical care but did not spare us the indignities, frustrations, and waste of time imposed by the current depersonalization of healthcare. In prior chapters, I have commented on the frustration of trying to reach a physician, the long waiting times on a telephone call, the never-ending conversations with robots and even less helpful individuals, the inability to maintain a relationship with a particular doctor, the absence of choice of a physician, and the limitations of available therapies. My family and I have participated in these impositions of today's healthcare.

I have related the story of hip replacement surgery in a five-star, world renowned, institution where the orthopedic surgeon, too busy doing multiple surgeries, did not bother to see the patient before or after surgery, indeed, on the entire day of surgery.

A friend's daughter believed that she had a close relationship with a particular obstetrician who saw her for all her prenatal visits. However, that individual did not deliver her baby or even come to see her during her hospital stay, because she was not "assigned" to the in-patient service at that time. The obstetrician did not even walk across the street from the clinic to say, "Hello," to *her* patient during 16 hours of labor or the 2-day post-partem stay. I have previously mentioned the true story of a doctor charging $25 for a letter stating a patient's ill health during the COVID-19 crisis.

As for myself, I have been riding horses since I was a boy. For the first time in my life, at age 83, I was bucked off a horse in 2016 at a ranch in Tucson. I broke eleven ribs on my right side, four in two places, sustained a comminuted fracture of the right scapula, and, in addition, had a hemothorax, a contused lung, with my heart pushed slightly to the left, and a blood loss from 15.6 to 11.6 g/dL. I was taken to the nearest hospital by ambulance and spent 7 h in the Emergency Room *without care* until the first hospitalist to see me passed me on to the next-in-line hospitalist, who admitted me to the monitored, intensive care, step-down unit for the next 18 days. There I was seen by different hospitalists daily. I was never introduced to the head of the unit, if there was one.

While in this unit, I was visited by several consulting cardiologists and pulmonologists, only when they decided to look in on me and not when I requested a visit. I was a metric in the files, database, and statics of the private company, the firm, that owned the hospital. I was often misdiagnosed, given the wrong drugs or dosage, had complications that were totally avoidable, and was denied essential respiratory care until acting as my own doctor I insisted upon it. Members of my family took shifts, day and night, never leaving me alone, to protect and to advocate for me. They kept records of my medicines and often prevented me from being overdosed or underdosed, and they maintained a continual watch on my oxygen saturation. For real medical care, I consulted by phone with an intensive care physician in Minneapolis in the evenings and received sound medical advice through visits and telephone conversations with another trusted physician friend.

Interestingly, the care I received shifted to the positive during the next 15 days of my 33-day hospitalization when I was transferred to the rehabilitation unit. This section of the hospital was well staffed and under the care of an older physician, a hold-over from the time when this hospital was owned by a religious order, a not-for-profit facility.

The New World

Virtual patient visits were becoming a reality prior to COVID-19; during COVID-19 they became the norm. Healthcare has embraced the virtual world. In doing so, we are obligated to make this system work not only for the providers of healthcare but for our patients as well. Long-range robotic surgery can bring skills and technology to far-removed people and places. Virtual patient-doctor visits, if properly staffed, can enhance frequency of communication and help to rekindle the intimacy of patient care. By restricting or eliminating the physical space for in-person visits, healthcare may become less expensive as well.

In every time of stress and upheaval, some individuals and institutions profit from the situation, and often new societal concepts are introduced.

One such innovation is "concierge medicine," or "retainer medicine," a growing concept in the USA. Concierge medicine is a fee-for-service business model, in which patients pay monthly or annual membership fees to have accessibility to a single physician, on-call, 24/7. For the patient, concierge medicine is, in a sense, a return to the doctor/patient relationship—at an extra financial cost. The system creates a separate tier of healthcare for those who can afford it. In the past, the very wealthy could always enjoy concierge medicine; now the upper middle class can do so as well. Concierge medicine is highly profitable for the participating physician. The average annual retainer fee is $3500, and the average number of clients is 250, making the annual concierge medicine practice revenue $850,000. In addition, the physician can bill insurance companies for services that can be reimbursed. We, the American people, must ask ourselves if adding the tier of concierge medicine to our national healthcare is moral in a society that voices the belief that universal healthcare is a right not a privilege.

Another innovation, again at an out-of-pocket cost, is hiring a professional agency to counteract the clerical, robot, and personal wall separating the patient from actual healthcare. These companies are the personal equivalent of the clerical forces hired by clinics, hospitals, and medical practices to navigate the business management of today's healthcare. These agencies will obtain your medical records, make your medical appointments, assemble your laboratory data, etc. In essence, they serve as a personal medical assistant, saving the customer service time and aggravation. For convenience, the product of this service is neatly packaged for the consumer on his/her iPhone.

Advertising directly to the patient via the media, in particular TV, capitalizes on the fractured doctor/patient relationship by suggesting drugs and therapy. All of us are now familiar with the TV commercial informing the viewer of an allegedly fantastic pharmaceutical or lifestyle program that will make a patient healthier, live longer, or combat a particular disease. The strong sell message is followed by a lightning-fast reading of every possible side effect of the advertised product, providing legal protection for the advertiser. If the commercial is for a drug available only by prescription, the commercial ends by telling the listener to discuss the product with their doctor. Often the commercial ends with a contact phone number and/or an email address. Such advertising campaigns are covert sabotage of the doctor/patient relationship. The media message implies that the advertiser knows more than the doctor, especially concerning recent medical advances. The commercial suggests that the viewer should tell the doctor what to prescribe. There is no better example of healthcare upside down than healthcare profiteers instructing potential customers on the advantages of their products, bypassing the nation's trained physicians, and assuming ownership of medical counseling.

My Doctor, My Patient

"My" as a determinant, pronoun, or adjective is used to indicate possession. The possession implied in "my doctor," or "my patient," does not, however, connate ownership, but stands for an association predicated on trust, respect, and caring.

When the patient says, "my doctor," he/she conveys trust in the judgment and good intentions of the doctor, in the doctor's ability to understand the patient's problems and provide the best available therapy. Ultimately, the patient verbalizes trust in the doctor by using the possessive "my" designation.

When the doctor says, "my patient," he/she is not boasting of, or taking pride in, a form of possession, as an indication of professional reputation and acumen. The doctor is voicing trust, respect, and possibly affection for the individual patient. The doctor trusts the patient to be honest in allowing the doctor the intimacy of knowledge necessary for the doctor to be of service. By assuming this responsibility, the doctor assumes an obligation. The doctor respects the patient as an individual in need of unbiased help. Over time, in some cases, this mutuality of trust engenders affection; the patient becomes a friend.

Conclusions

In the world of the modern clinic, hospital, and the medical practice taught in today's medical schools, the patient enters the realm of the firm, provider/employees administering to clients, devoid of a personal relationship, under an administocracy. It is impossible to speak of "my" doctor or "my" patient, if the actors in the drama of healthcare are interchangeable, impersonal, and, essentially, anonymous.

The ultimate foundation of healthcare is based on the doctor/patient relationship. If we eliminate the mutual "my," we no longer have healthcare for individual human beings.

Sources

Chipidza FE, et al. Impact of the doctor-patient relationship. Prim Care Companion CNS Disord. 2015;17(5):1840. https://doi.org/10.4088/PCC.15f01840.

Definitive Healthcare. What Is concierge medicine? https://www.definitivehc.com/blog/what-is-concierge-medicine

Kaba R, Sooriakumaran P. The evolution of the doctor-patient relationship. Int J Surg. 2007;5(1):57–65. https://doi.org/10.1016/j.ijsu.2006.01.005.

Kirk L. Professionalism in medicine: definitions and considerations for teaching. Proc Bayl Univ Med Cent. 2007;20(1):13–6. https://doi.org/10.1080/08998280.2007.11928225.

Chapter 14
Where Do We Go from Here?

> *Evil is not to be traced back to the individual but to the*
> *collective behavior of humanity.*
>
> *Reinhold Niebuhr, American Theologian, 1892-1971*

A Story

But the emperor has nothing at all on!

"Listen to the voice of innocence!" exclaimed his father; and what the child had said was whispered from one to another.

"But he has nothing at all on!" at last cried all the people.

The emperor was vexed, for he suspected they were right. But he thought, "This procession has got to go on." So he walked more proudly than ever, as his noblemen held high the train that wasn't there at all.

"The Emperor's New Clothes," Hans Christian Andersen, 1837

Reinhold Niebuhr, American theologian, President of the Union Theological Seminary in New York City, was one of my teachers during my elective year as an undergraduate at Columbia College. He is the author of what has been designated the Serenity Prayer: *God, grant me the serenity to accept the things I cannot change, the courage to change the things I can, and the wisdom to know the difference.*

Niebuhr certainly believed that evil individuals existed (e.g., Hitler), but that the greater perpetration of evil required collective behavior. In classroom discussions, he brought this philosophy down to everyday life by stating his distrust of committee decisions, wherein no one assumed responsibility. He preferred placing the authority for the stipulation of principles and key interventions in the hands of an independent individual. He firmly believed in the morality of one over the ethos of a conglomerate. This concept has been the underlying precept in the prior chapters demonstrating today's healthcare dominated by a self-perpetuating administocracy, whether by a top-down chain-of-command structure, interchangeable healthcare providers, the loss of trust by a fractured doctor/patient relationship, or of healthcare by industry—in essence, Healthcare Upside Down.

The story excerpt from Hans Christian Andersen's 1837 tale of "The Emperor's New Clothes" has three take-aways: (1) It may take one voice to point out what is truly obvious to all. (2) The perpetrators of an illusion will maintain that deception even when it is shown to be false. (3) The child who cried *"But the emperor has nothing at all on!"* was not required to make a suit of clothes for the emperor. In this book, I have tried to give voice to what is obvious—our healthcare is upside down and Americans are not getting their money's worth. The parties responsible for this state of affairs profit from it and will not change it but will continue to maintain this system.

Turning healthcare right-side up cannot be left to a single segment of the community. It will require intensive thought and action by: (1) healthcare workers and their leadership, (2) the advocates of public health, (3) the medical schools of our nation, (4) medical and social researchers, (5) insurers of healthcare, (6) hospital and clinical providers, (7) government and politicians, (8) the media, (9) philanthropy, and (10) every taxpayer and beneficiary.

Ten Potential Remedies

Healthcare Workers and Their Leadership

This remedy requires above all the willingness to band together and to assume leadership. When I speak of healthcare workers, I refer to physicians, nurse practitioners, nurses, orderlies, ambulance drivers, and all those others who play vital roles in the daily delivery of healthcare to their fellow citizens. It is essential that they first and foremost be part of this remedy.

Many physicians would prefer to continue the current healthcare system; they are pleased with the lifestyle it offers them. They have willingly sacrificed their professional liberty for prescribed hours of service, more family and recreation time, a planned retirement, and the limitation of responsibility offered by the dissolution of the doctor/patient relationship. They prefer shared patients and a fixed income. In essence, they choose to be service employees. Even if they harbor an attraction for individualism, freedom of choice, and autonomy, these concepts have been subjugated to a prescribed life: a job. These same physicians, however, may be persuaded to join the ranks of healthcare workers attempting to change healthcare if it becomes expedient for them to do so in order to maintain their membership in our profession.

I call upon those physicians who share my view of the practice of medicine enumerated throughout this book, to say, "Enough is enough, we must reestablish the healthcare concept embodied by the doctor/patient relationship." Going back in time is never feasible. It is, however, possible to incorporate what was worthwhile in the past to create the future. The purpose of history is to provide guidelines and lessons. A group of like-minded physicians can provide the guidance and the example for affirmative changes in the medical schools, clinics, hospitals, and practices discussed in prior chapters. Individual physicians working together can challenge the system and the administocracy in charge of the system.

It is essential that these leaders assume advocacy roles within, and make these goals intrinsic to the mission of, their leadership organizations, e.g., the American Medical Association, the American College of Physicians, the American College of Surgeons, etc. These organizations are our unions of commonality; they have outreach; they have money; and they speak to politicians, the media, and the public. They, unlike the individual protestor, are less vulnerable to retaliation. These organizations represent one-half of the doctor/patient relationship. It is with these groups that healthcare reform must start.

Advocates of Public Health

In the final analysis, concern with the health of individuals becomes public health and falls into the domain of the officers of our national Public Health Service and its eight huge divisions. They are the national source of healthcare information and healthcare guidelines. They are the advocates for the public good. They directly influence the 60–65% of socialized medicine practiced in our nation. They have the monetary and organizational support of the US government, to whom they report.

And therein lies a problem: these advocates of healthcare report to politicians who may choose to regulate public healthcare pronouncements, as was so vividly exemplified in the tragic US failure in responding to the COVID-19 pandemic.

In November 2020, the American Surgical Association (ASA), the oldest (established in 1880) and probably the most conservative body of American surgeons issued an ASA Council policy statement. The text of this statement, published in the *Annals of Surgery*, is short and unambiguous:

> The foundation of the achievements of modern medicine, including surgery, has been the scientific method. Unfortunately, there is a growing pattern in US politics to discredit science. The American Surgical Association, as the leading body of surgical scientists, stands in solidarity with other scientists to condemn such attacks. Objective scientific facts should not be suppressed as a political tool. While science should be used to inform politics, we firmly believe that politics should not dictate science. How to act upon scientific facts can be a legitimate part of political debate. The existence of scientific facts should not be. We call upon our members, all surgeons, and health care workers of all political beliefs to confront anti-science attitudes and attacks that have become part of our political discourse.

The advocates of public health must be guided by research-derived facts not opinion, wishful thinking, or the next national election. Regardless of who issues their paychecks, their responsibility, the job of public health doctors, is to act as believable authorities, warranting public respect and adherence to their recommendations. Above all, they must be servants of science, unfettered in their public role as independent national healthcare spokespersons. They may work for a government agency, but their moral duty is to serve the citizens of the nation. They must be true to their calling to prevent and to cure disease.

Medical Schools

Healthcare begins in the medical schools of our nation. What is taught to emerging doctors during the four formal years of schooling and subsequent years of residency training, by didactics and by example, is the blueprint for the future of healthcare.

There have been eras in the history of medical schools and teaching institutions that have propelled healthcare into new dimensions, that have been the progenitors of concepts and innovations for vanquishing diseases and promoting increased human health. In fairly modern times, two epochs of surgical innovations are exemplars: The Halsted era at John's Hopkins Hospital, in Baltimore, 1890–1922, and the Wangensteen era at the University of Minnesota, in Minneapolis, 1938–1967.

William Stuart Halsted introduced strict aseptic techniques in the operating room, new anesthetics, and several new procedures, including the radical mastectomy for breast cancer. His everlasting achievement, however, was in organizing, in association with William Osler, in medicine, Howard Kelly in Gynecology, and William Welch in Pathology, the modern residency program, that stimulated generations of surgical pioneers, including the great neurosurgeon, Harvey Cushing.

I wrote a book about the Wangensteen era in Minnesota that illustrates what can be done in healthcare and how to achieve it (Surgical Renaissance in the Heartland: A Memoir of the Wangensteen Era, University of Minnesota Press, 2020). During the long tenure of Owen H. Wangensteen as Chair of Surgery, the foundation for open-heart procedures, heart and pancreas transplantation, bariatric/obesity surgery, implantable infusion pump therapies, and other medical landmarks originated and forever changed medicine and the lives of millions. Wangensteen, like Halsted, attracted a generation of like-minded physicians who thrived in an atmosphere of debate, the unfettered expression of ideas, and the opportunities to research their imaginative concepts. This engine of productivity turned out 38 department heads, 31 division heads, 72 directors of surgical programs, and 110 full professors who subsequently empowered many of the medical schools in our nation.

In this enterprise, Wangensteen, for the most part, was supported by the deans and senior administration of the University of Minnesota. They were cognizant of the opportunity offered by this group of physicians, with their mid-western and western roots, to raise the University of Minnesota above the status of a state medical school, fairly unrecognized and ignored by the big-name schools of the East, South, and California. Indeed, the Wangensteen era propelled the University of Minnesota not only to global recognition but to global acclaim.

Contrary to the above examples, the integrity of medical schools throughout the country by the late 1990s has been threatened or destroyed by the rise of imperial administration, the administocracy described in Chap. 3. No longer is freedom of action and thought by the faculty encouraged but it is actively suppressed. The illustrative stories of Chap. 3 demonstrate how deans and presidents now expected obeisant behavior by faculty and philanthropic donors, primarily concerned with maintaining top-down leadership of unquestioned acquiescence. They, like Hans Christian Andersen's emperor, continue to uphold the grandeur of their invisible new clothes, and, to them, dissidents are not fit for their jobs and should be removed. If administocracy is not stymied, the words of Andersen's truth-telling child will go unheeded. At this time, however, autocratic medical school administocracy is becoming dominant throughout our country.

The remedies I would suggest to heal medical schools are two-fold and best instituted simultaneously: (1) restoration of strong departments within the medical school and (2) installing administrations who facilitate, not dictate.

In the time of Wangensteen and others, clinical departments and their chairs were responsible for patient care in their discipline, teaching, research, and faculty remuneration. Today, in many medical schools, patient care by the department's physicians is in a service line that reports not to the department chair but to the dean via a service-line associate dean. For example, a faculty surgeon is no longer responsible for his/her surgical performance to a chair of surgery but to a dean, who is unlikely ever to have been a surgeon. Clinical teaching now depends on the service-line clinical experience. Research orientation is now not primarily the choice of the member of the faculty but is supervised, controlled, and possibly mandated by the chair of a department, acting under instructions of the dean. Faculty income has been removed from departmental discretion and is under the jurisdiction of an independent practice-plan group, of which, once again, the dean is in charge. In other words, the chair of a medical school department is a chair in name only, reduced in authority to the role of a figurehead under the rule of the dean and central administration.

Can a single department of like-minded individuals, with a charismatic leader, resist these institutional impositions? Probably not, if acting alone. I have known of one such attempt where a superb department of anesthesia said "no" to becoming employees of an outstanding pediatric hospital. The administration of that hospital severed its relationship with the group and hired more compliant anesthesiologists. Nevertheless, the courage to deny subjugation of departments must come from within our medical schools, from professors protected by tenure from being fired, and, to be successful, should involve a multi-departmental effort.

Can resistance to administocracy come from within the administrations themselves? It is unlikely that as a body, or by the actions of a few individuals, today's system would foster the demise of administrative imperialism. Yet, visionary new leaders might emerge from faculty ranks, remember their roots and traditions, and be motivated to initiate change.

As I emphasized in Chap. 3 on medical schools, nearly everyone in the nation pays directly or indirectly for the education of their doctors. Thus, the public has a stake in the nation's medical schools; the public needs to have its voice heard on how their doctors are educated and trained. Healthcare starts with the doctor/trainee. Therefore, the healthcare of individual members of the public, and the public as a whole, starts with the ethos and schooling of public-supported medical schools. The proper education of the young is the best way to supplant the entrenched, poorly functioning precepts of the current healthcare structure.

Medical and Social Research

Medical research, based on the scientific method, generally starts with a need and works towards eliminating that need with a new discovery—an insight, a principle, a method, a device. A primary source of medical research is the medical school, however, industry and government not only finance but perform research. Common to all research, as previously discussed, is freedom of thought and the financial support to investigate. For research to promote progress, its results and the knowledge gained must be granted open dissemination.

Modern research requires big data and the employment of sophisticated computer analyses. Today's healthcare analysts are dedicated to this science. Their endeavors collate pandemic data, derive precise statistics, and based on varying assumptions, predict the timing of pandemic outcomes. These same systems can analyze our current healthcare variables and offer outcome projections for current or alternative concepts. Clinical data input for these analyses can be derived from polling public opinion. In this respect, societal research includes the all-important input of members of society in formulating healthcare remedies for society.

Insurers of Healthcare

Looking to the insurers of healthcare for remedies to current healthcare necessitates looking at two extremes—socialized medicine and the entrepreneurs of insurance.

Socialized medicine offers certain advantages but many offsetting disadvantages (Chap. 8). Consideration of socialized medicine as a remedy raises several questions: Can governments offer efficient and beneficial healthcare? Can some governments do this better than others? Can our government do this? Can there exist a working coalition of socialized and private sector healthcare that best serves the public? In discussing US healthcare objectively, not influenced by inflammatory accusations or inaccurate interpretations and perceptions, we need to remember that US healthcare is currently 60–65% socialized medicine in principle, some of it functioning very well, some not so well. As a nation, what aspects of socialized medicine do we wish to keep and what do we reject? To make these choices, we must examine outcomes and not be influenced by pejorative language and unexamined prejudices.

The private, for-profit healthcare insurance system serves its stockholders in the marketplace and not its stakeholders of insurees. Certainly, the CEOs and the other members of the administration of these companies will not voluntarily surrender their astronomical incomes. These fiscal privileges of the very few are the result of limited, expensive services to the many. Government intercession may provide some rectification, but in the free economy we espouse to represent, the alternative to current healthcare insurance is competition; a free and transparent competition that provides equal or better service, with fewer limitations, at a lower price.

I believe this competition can be provided in the private sector by not-for-profit institutions. Many exist today but often function as limited fraternal organizations, e.g. American Postal Workers Union, or regional chapters, e.g., Blue Cross/Blue Shield. These companies need to broaden their clientele and coalesce nationally. For example, the United Services Automobile Association (USAA) was funded in 1922 by 25 Army officers to provide automobile self-insurance. Membership was rapidly extended to all active and retired officers and enlisted members of the Armed Forces, as well as their families. The USAA portfolio further expanded to offer a full range of insurance services. As a private, reciprocal, non-profit, inter-insurance exchange it has become a Fortune 500 company with thirteen million members. USAA profits are distributed to insured stakeholders.

The private health insurance business is fertile ground for fiscal entrepreneurs. By cutting administrative personnel and their exorbitant incomes, coupled with offering superior patient services and returning profits to their insured clients, old and new not-for-profits should be competitive with the for-profits. The National Committee for Quality Assurance (NCQA), a non-profit healthcare accreditation and quality measurement group ranks 474 private plans, obtained through employment or self-insurance. The number one ranked private plan was the not-for-profit Harvard Pilgrim Health Care's HMO in New England. The not-for-profit plans as a group ranked higher than the for-profit ones.

A suggested remedy for healthcare within the current insurance industry is for the purchaser to research the selection of their insurance company. The self-employed, self-insured can freely do this. What about the large segment of the population insured via policies selected by their employers? The "middlemen" in this process may consider cost above benefit value. They may select an insurance firm that offers the company a cheaper group policy by specifically omitting a service, e.g., obesity healthcare. The remedy here is for employee unions, or individual employees, to voice their insurance preference. In doing so they need to protect all the people in their group, with all diseases and disabilities. In insurance purchases, the policy holder hopes not to be one of the winners, the person who gets sick or dies; the purchaser is buying peace of mind for themselves, their families, and the working group they belong to.

Providers: Hospitals and Clinics

A massive effort for the restoration of the doctor/patient relationship, with all of its implications, from doctors and other healthcare workers, researchers, medical schools, and by a revamped insurance industry, will force hospitals and clinics to listen. The robot inquisitors will diminish, the staff will be more hospitable, the patient's wishes will be respected, and patients will have care relationships with identifiable physicians. These changes may not be altruistic in origin of intent but adopted for survival in a world of competition. Thus, the remedy to turn hospital and clinical healthcare right-side up will take outside pressure, essentially, the will of the people who pay for their healthcare.

Government and Politicians

Essentially every US institution of government, executive, legislative, judicial, has made healthcare a partisan issue, an unfortunate situation. Members of all political parties, from every social economic stratum, within the full range of diversity, need healthcare at one time or another. The governance of healthcare should, therefore, be a common concern of all branches of government, uncontaminated by political allegiances. Only then we will achieve true national healthcare, true American healthcare, devoid of pejorative labeling.

Another aspect of our US government planning, financing, and administrating healthcare has been the practice, by whichever political party is in the majority, of not fully consulting the healthcare profession before enacting laws. I am certain that prior to an infrastructure bill that includes repairing old and building new bridges is written, bridge engineers are consulted. It has not, however, been the routine in our national practice to consult and work with life-long healthcare professionals and their organizations in formulating healthcare legislation.

From the smallest town of our nation to the running of our federal government, lawyers are in charge. Presidential Cabinet appointments to the post of Secretary of Health and Human Services have been, for the most part, lawyers, not doctors. If it were customary to make similar appointments to people outside of their field of expertise, the Attorney General of the United States should not be a lawyer but from another profession. Federal laws have never impinged on the right of lawyers to charge whatever they chose and to perform pro bono services. Yet, there are several laws on the book, regulating doctors' fees and making pro bono work by a doctor actually a crime (Chap. 6). Our public servants, therefore, seem to take aim at doctors, one-half of the doctor/patient relationship of healthcare.

Everyone is, at one time or another, a patient. It is, therefore, patients who vote the lawyers (who are also patients) into office. We, the patients, must tell our elected, and want-to-be-elected, lawyers, what we desire for our healthcare and that our vote is contingent on their representing that perspective. This remedy of a free society can be carried out in a variety of ways by advocacy, and most successfully by paid lobbyists. Nearly all of us as citizens belong to some large, powerful union with a professional group of lawyer lobbyists, e.g., National Education Association of the United States, 2,731,416 members; Teamsters, 1,400,000 members. Our lobbyists must be instructed to advocate to government, industry, and all aspects of healthcare for the healthcare we want and pay for.

The Media

The role of the media is to present news, to entertain, and to provide commentary. To be trusted, the media must not fabricate (e.g., assign political ideals or religious beliefs to a biochemical viral entity, devoid of the basic definition of life, the ability of self-reproduction) or lie (e.g., state that a face mask does not offer protection from particle infection by the wearer and from the wearer). Media is communication. It can communicate the statistics of healthcare and our national failings; it can offer a dialogue for proposed remedies; it can empower voices of reason and the will of the majority. Today's media often profits in controversy. There certainly exists controversy in combating the forces that promote the current state of healthcare by giving voice to its opponents. Today, the combined media in all of its manifestations are a powerful force in changing the dynamics of society. In making people aware that healthcare is upside down but can be righted, and that we are all being defrauded, the media can be an ally.

Philanthropy

The US standard of living has been greatly enhanced by the charitable donations of philanthropy. Today, billions of dollars are given annually for healthcare: direct or indirect patient services, infrastructure, development of new therapeutic approaches, and basic research.

Those of us who are interested in rectifying the US healthcare system must educate individual philanthropists and philanthropic organizations that the current healthcare system needs to change its orientation if we are to reverse our dismal US statistics in world healthcare ranking from that of a third-world, or near third-world, nation (Chap. 1). A major billionaire funder, or a large philanthropic organization, could fund a program to alter those statistics over time. Today's wealthiest Americans earn billions of dollars annually and give away billions; these individuals could finance such an enterprise. Existing fraternal groups might create an effective, if odd-ball alliance, to fund this effort, e.g., the American Surgical Association and the Teamsters. After all, the healthcare goals of their members are identical—to offer their families, and our nation, individuals and institutions, a system that embodies science, honesty, security, trust, and humanity.

Everyone

Everyone, meaning nearly the entire US population, pays for healthcare outright, via purchased insurance, or by tax-based government support. In one way or another, this money comes out of everyone's earnings or savings. The over 60% socialized medicine programs of this country, such as Medicare and Medicaid, are directly funded by taxpayers.

Each citizen is, therefore, a consumer making a purchase. Is it not time for the totally essential purchase of healthcare to involve customer preference? The average car shopper looks at several brands and models; the average clothes buyer compares value and price; even the average consumer of basics such as food examines groceries before buying them. Yet, today, the average patient may grumble but accepts interminable robotic calls to a healthcare provider, impersonal medical care, mandated therapy, being ordered to vacate a hospital bed while still in pain, and many more indignities. Above all, everyone has accepted the dissolution of the time-honored, cherished doctor/patient relationship. The only exceptions are the very few ultrarich who are content with the system because they can afford to opt out of it. Many of them also derive enormous personal incomes from this paradox.

The remedy to fix healthcare upside down, the remedy that encompasses all the other remedies suggested, is the raised voice of the people—the actual consumer of healthcare. All responsible members of society need to decide whether they are satisfied with their current system as analyzed in these pages, or if they wish to use their right of self-determination to alter the system to what they, as the ultimate buyer, wish to purchase. To achieve affirmative change, the voices of individuals, leadership organizations, educators and researchers, entrepreneur insurers, politicians, a receptive media, and philanthropic institutions must be heard. As stated in Chap. 2, language is the transformative precursor of reality.

Conclusions

Where do we go from here? Each individual member of our society as a healthcare consumer needs to learn what she/he is purchasing with tax or out-of-pocket dollars. Though some of the purchases may be excellent, much of it could be improved. In far too many aspects, healthcare today is not consumer friendly. To achieve affirmative change—to turn healthcare right-side up—is the responsibility of individuals working through all their available affiliations. The will of the people must be heard by government and private initiatives if healthcare is to truly serve the people.

Sources

Azar AM, et al. Reforming America's healthcare system through choice and competition. https://www.hhs.gov/sites/default/files/Reforming-Americas-Healthcare-System-Through-Choice-and-Competition.pdf.

Harris PA. Health reform: how to improve US. health care in 2020 and beyond. 2019. https://www.ama-assn.org/about/leadership/health-reform-how-improve-us-health-care-2020-and-beyond.

PWC. The empowered consumer. https://www.pwc.com/healthcare.

Rosenthal E. An American sickness: how healthcare became big business and how you can take it back. New York: Penguin Press; 2017.

Tabri ZA. Health insurance – for-profit vs nonprofit. 2020. https://medium.com/beingwell/health.

Epilogue

Healthcare is an integral function of a society. It is fair to state that the inalienable rights proclaimed in our Declaration of Independence of life, liberty, and the pursuit of happiness are encompassed in healthcare. Before, during, and maybe even more so after COVID-19, US healthcare has become a depersonalized business, profitable for a very few, paid for by the majority. Healthcare has negated freedom of choice of medical care, caregiver, and, often, therapeutic options. Healthcare pro bono and financial patient courtesy have been made illegal; indeed, healthcare is practiced without any courtesy whatsoever. Healthcare is practiced without personal independence by patients and physicians, under the top-down dominance of a ruling administocracy. US healthcare statistics are inferior to essentially those of every comparable nation, at a monetary cost well above that of every nation on earth.

The opening moment of life—birth—involves healthcare for mother and child. Growing up and achieving adulthood involves healthcare. Being able to live a mature life, to work, to love, to have children is dependent on healthcare. And, the final chapter, aging, can be realized and even made pleasurable by healthcare. Healthcare is, therefore, integral to life, from beginning to end. Healthcare is not a commodity but a necessity. Healthcare needs to be treated with respect. The establishment, practice, and financing of healthcare affect everyone, should not be neglected by anyone, and must be the concern of all of us.

I have been a doctor for sixty years, and during those years at times I have also been a patient. I have held the hands of my patients; I have been the one whose hand has been held. I have received trust and given trust. The therapeutic decisions my patients and I reached were not subject to the interdiction of a third party. I do not want to have my life's role as a physician and surgeon, my joy in the process, usurped by an administocracy. As a patient, I do not want to hold hands with a robot and confide my health problems to a faceless entity. As a doctor, a patient, a person, I reject the currently shattered doctor/patient relationship.

Healthcare is upside down. Let us set it right-side up.

H. Buchwald, *Healthcare Upside Down*, https://doi.org/10.1007/978-3-031-07163-8

Index

A
Adams, G., 53, 55
Adams, J., 80, 89
Administocracy, 16–18
Aetna, 53
Affordable Care Act (ACA), 62, 74
African Americans, 75
Agency for Healthcare Research and Equality
(AHRQ), 80
Agency for Toxic Substances and Disease
Registry (ATSDR), 80
Amazon, 53
American Medical Association (AMA), 36
AmerisourceBergen Corporation, 57
Andersen, H.C., 108, 111
Anti-vaxxers, 82
Antonine Plague, 83
Apgar, V., 77
Apple, 53
Aristotle, 94
Asian Americans, 76
Assuming responsibility, 45
Avian Flu, 83
Ayurveda, 70

B
Bacon, F., 72, 94
Bakken, E., 96
Berkshire Hathaway, 53
Blackburn, H., 79

Black Death, 83
Blake, Q., 33–40
Blue Cross/Blue Shield (BC/BS)
Associates, 52, 53
Boudreaux, G., 53
Bourla, A., 56
Bramante, 34
Bretolini, M., 53
Broussard, B.D., 53
Bundling costs, 36, 37
Burnout, 23, 24
Bush, G.H.W., 69
Business model, 30

C
Callender, D.L., 55
Care Conference, 14
Centers for Disease Control and Prevention
(CDC), 88, 89
Chain-of-command structure, 16, 20
Champy, J., 17
Cleanliness, 80
Client, 15
The clinic, 29–32, 114
Cocoliztli Epidemic, 83
Compartmentalization of responsibility, 39
Computer algorithms, 30
Concierge medicine, 104
Consumer Reports magazine, 62
Cook, M., 20